ALWAYS BEEN ME.

HOME NOW.

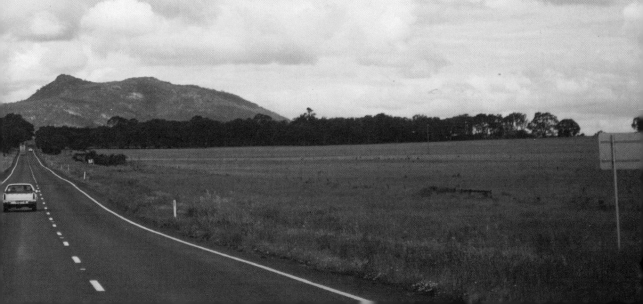

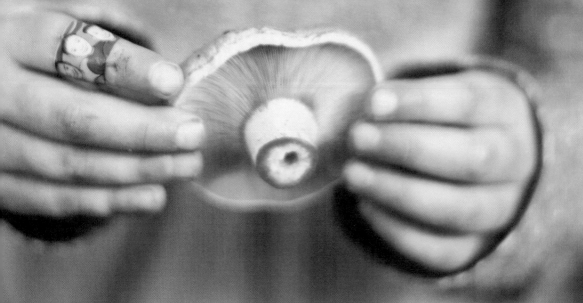

THIS IS THE GOOD LIFE, PEOPLE.

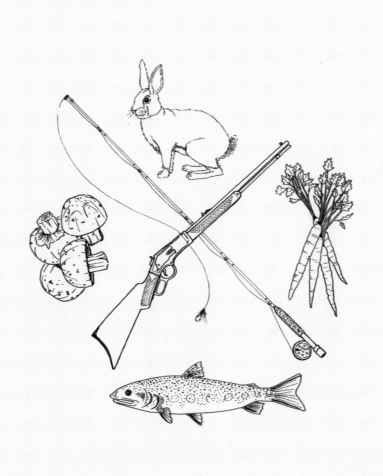

WHO

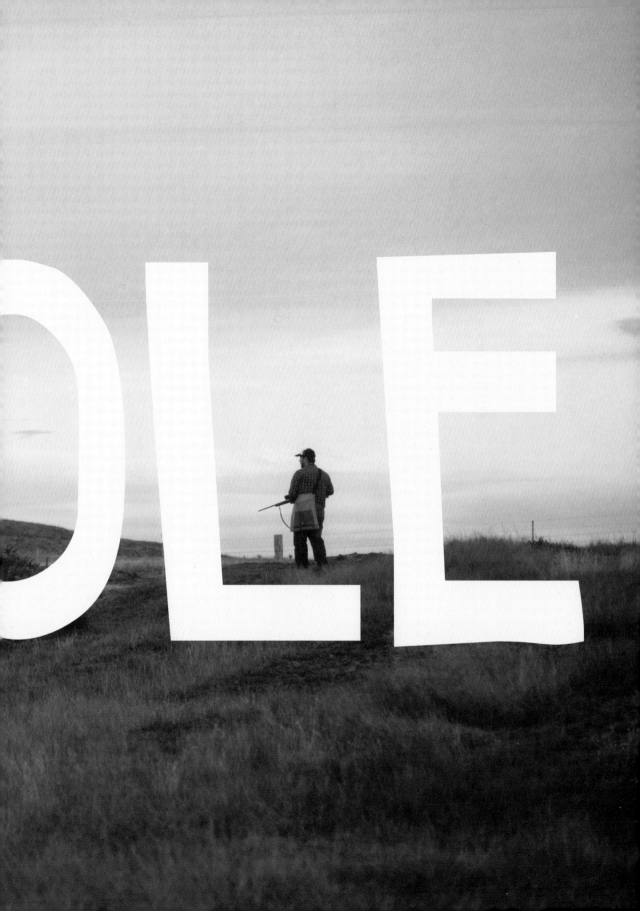

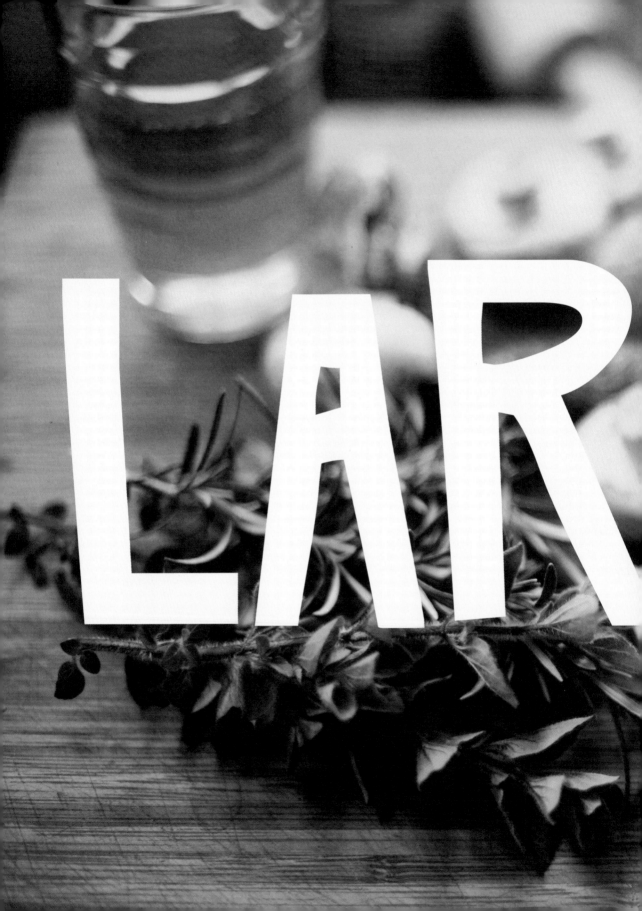

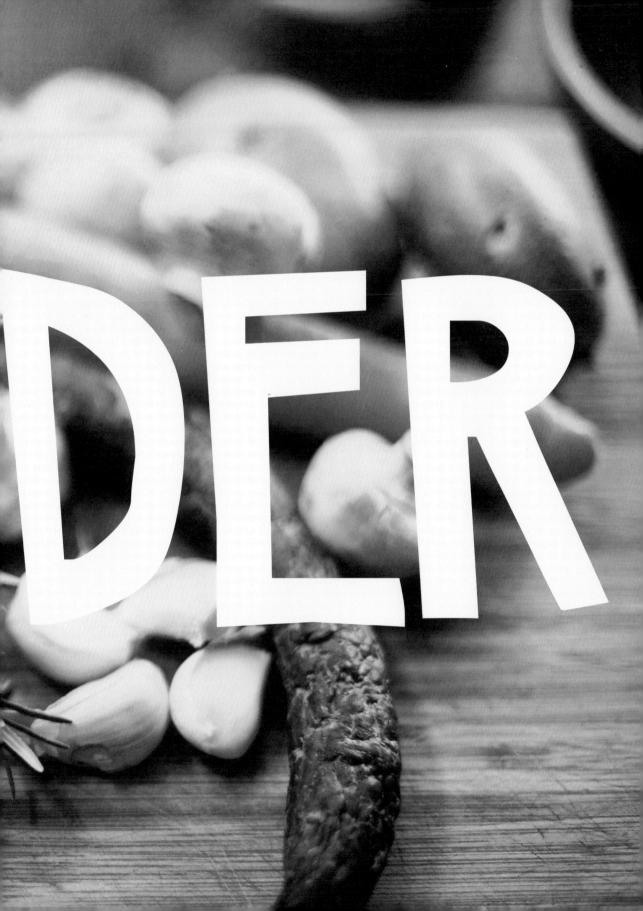

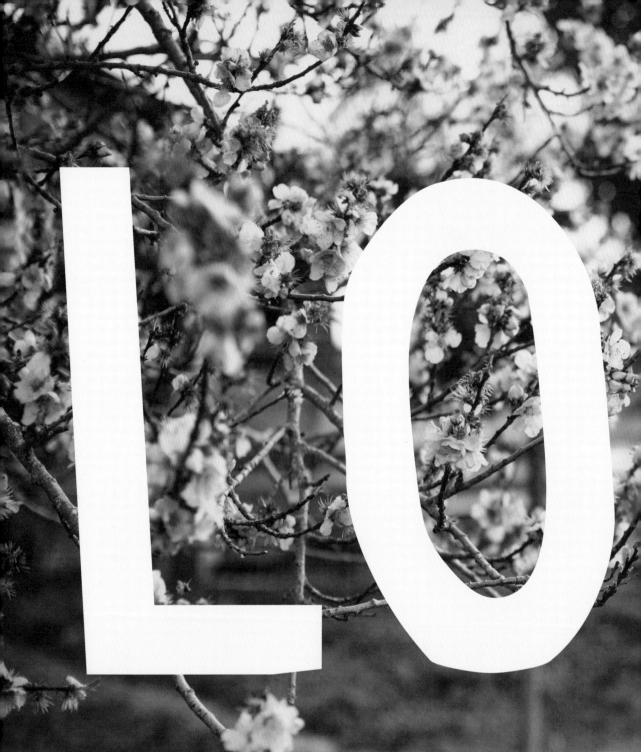

GROW • GATHER

 powerHouse Books
Brooklyn, NY

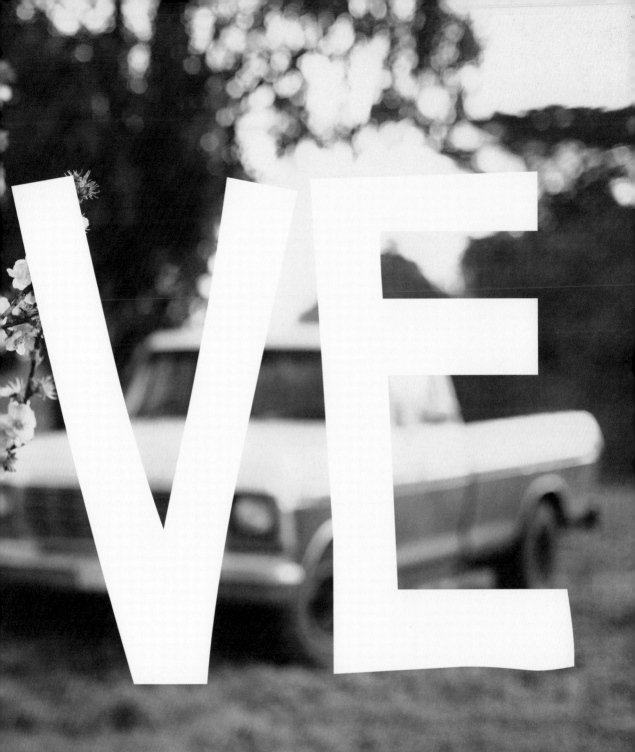

VE

HUNT · COOK

BY ROHAN ANDERSON

THERE IS A CONNECTIVITY OF THIS LIFE OF OURS.

I LIKE THAT IT'S COMPLEX, THAT IT'S CONNECTED AND UNENDING, AND THAT ALL THINGS ARE LINKED BY SOME INVISIBLE THREAD. I LIKE THAT WE ARE FLAWED, THAT WE CAN SHINE, AND THAT WE MAKE MISTAKES. MAKING THIS BOOK WAS ALL OF THOSE THINGS AND MORE. IT'S BEEN QUITE AN ADVENTURE, AN EYE OPENING EXPERIENCE. UNTIL I SAT DOWN AND DOCUMENTED WHAT I WAS ACTUALLY DOING (IN REGARDS TO FOOD) I DIDN'T REALIZE HOW INTERCONNECTED MY SYSTEM WAS. LOOKING AT FOOD ON A LARGER SCALE IS AN INTIMIDATING TASK, BUT BREAKING IT DOWN INTO LITTLE SECTIONS MAKES THE IDEA OF IT ALL LESS DAUNTING. AND TAKING BACK A LITTLE BIT OF CONTROL OF WHERE YOUR FOOD IS PRODUCED MAKES LIFE TEND TOWARDS THE SIMPLE SIDE.

THAT'S THE IDEA ANYWAY. SIMPLE DOESN'T MEAN YOU DON'T PUT IN EFFORT OR THAT YOU JUST LAY BACK AND WATCH THINGS HAPPEN. SIMPLE CAN SOMETIMES MEAN MORE WORK, MORE PLANNING, AND EVEN MORE THOUGHT PUT INTO YOUR PHILOSOPHY OF LIFE. THE WORK COMES IN THE FORM OF GETTING SOIL UNDER YOUR FINGERNAILS, BLOOD ON YOUR SHIRT, AND BEADS OF SWEAT ON YOUR FOREHEAD COOKING OVER A HOT STOVE. THE PLANNING COMES IN THE FORM OF SEASONAL PREPARATIONS AND ANNUAL EVENTS THAT KEEP YOUR FOOD STORES IN CHECK AND YOUR VEGETABLE PATCH HAPPY AND PRODUCTIVE. AND FINALLY, BRINGING IT ALL TOGETHER, IS YOUR APPROACH TO LIFE IN GENERAL. MY PHILOSOPHY IS BASIC: NATURE RULES SUPREME. WE ARE ONLY LITTLE GEARS THAT MAKE THE BIGGER MACHINE DO ITS THING.

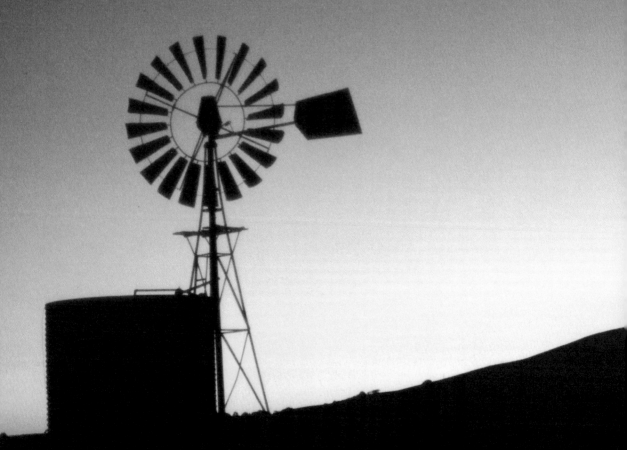

ALTHOUGH, FOOLS THAT WE ARE, AS A SPECIES WE OFTEN LIVE AS THOUGH WE ARE THE OPERATOR OF THE MACHINE.

A WARNING TO THOSE WHO ARE NOT REGULAR READERS OF MY BLOG: I HAVE ATTITUDE, I HAVE OPINIONS. TO BE ABLE TO POST THEM ON A WALL FOR PEOPLE TO READ IS A GREAT HONOR. TAKE THEM OR LEAVE THEM—THAT'S COOL WITH ME. I AM JUST GLAD TO BE ABLE TO OFFER SOME SORT OF ALTERNATIVE. IT'S NOT AN ALL-OR-NOTHING APPROACH. I'M FAR FROM PERFECT WHEN IT COMES TO FOOD. LIVING COMPLETELY ETHICALLY INVOLVES LIVING IN A CAVE, COLD, AND NO DOUBT RATHER NAKED. NOT MY CUP OF TEA REALLY. BUT TO BE ABLE TO MAKE SOME CHANGES IN OUR LIVES THAT CAN HAVE A POSITIVE IMPACT ON THE HEALTH OF OURSELVES AND OUR ENVIRONMENT IS A GOOD THING. THE MORE WE SIMPLIFY AND REDIRECT OUR EFFORTS TO ACTIVITIES THAT BENEFIT US AND OUR COMMUNITIES THE MORE WE WILL HELP CHANGE THIS MESSED UP WORLD OF OURS, AND HOPEFULLY LEAVE BEHIND FOR OUR CHILDREN A PLANET STILL WILD AND BEAUTIFUL. THAT'S REALLY WHAT IT'S ALL ABOUT, ISN'T IT?

I HOPE YOU ENJOY THE RECIPES AS MUCH AS I DO EATING THEM! EXPERIMENT AS MUCH AS YOU LIKE. FOOD IS ONE BIG ADVENTURE. AND THIS IS BY NO MEANS EVERYTHING YOU NEED TO KNOW OR NECESSARILY THE ONLY WAY TO APPROACH LIFE; BUT IT'S WHAT WORKS FOR ME. I'M SHARING MY FOOD STORY. THIS IS A BOOK FULL OF THINGS THAT I'VE LEARNED ALONG THE WAY, TRICKS THAT I'VE DISCOVERED BY MAKING MANY A MISTAKE, AND TIPS THAT I'VE PICKED UP FROM FRIENDS AND ELDERS. IT'S A STARTING BLOCK. THE REST IS UP TO YOU.

—ROHAN

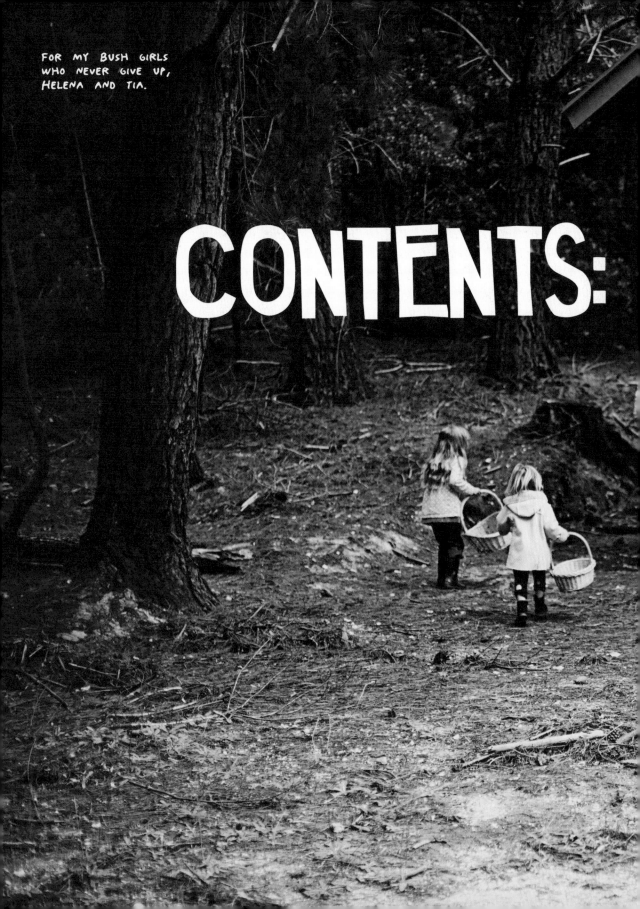

FOR MY BUSH GIRLS
WHO NEVER GIVE UP,
HELENA AND TIA.

CONTENTS:

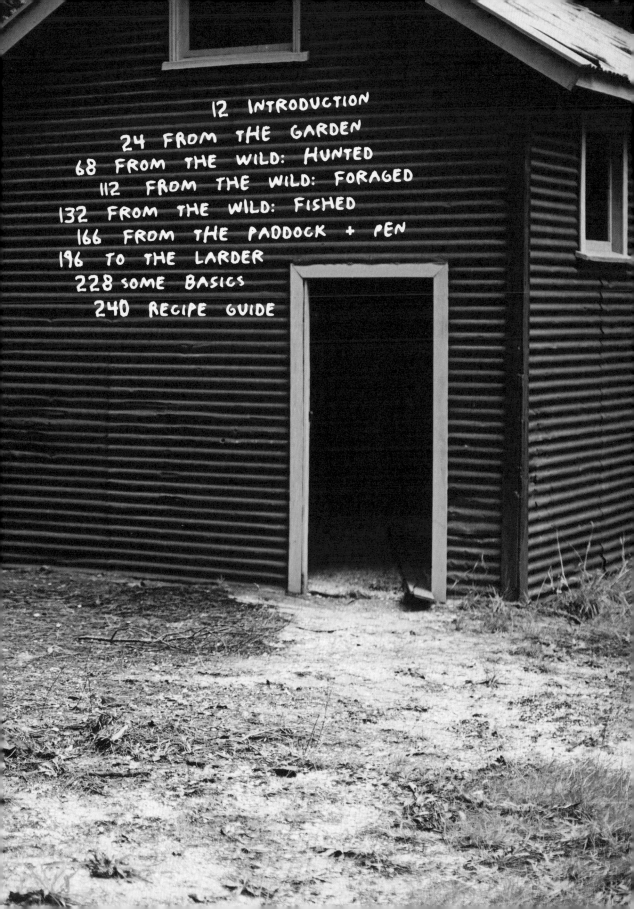

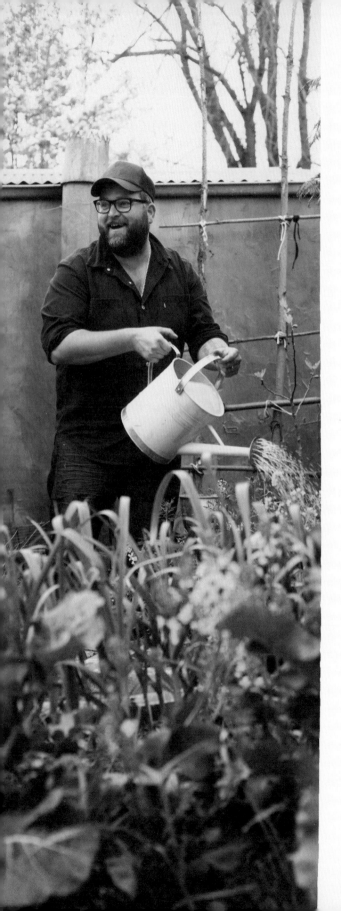

There are two basic ways to view food. On the one hand, it's merely a necessity for our survival, a source of energy to fuel our bodies. On the other (more exciting) hand, food can be appreciated for the indulgent pleasures of taste and texture. For many years I'd been content with these two understandings of food. That is, until I started studying natural resource management. I learned a great deal about the management, or more accurately the mismanagement, of our precious resources and consequently the current unhealthy state of the natural world. I started asking myself where my food came from and what impact my consumption of said food had on the world around me. The current age of broad-acre food production is undeniably flawed. The way that food is produced, shipped, and consumed globally has a negative impact on the environment, on our personal health, on local economies and communities, on our spiritual well-being, and on the quality and flavor of the food itself.

The most obvious and worrisome effect of our current industrialized method of food production, and what first got me to reexamine my own habits, was direct environmental damage: loss of biodiversity, soil degradation, habitat loss, and the damage caused by use of chemicals and pesticides, bioengineering, etc. One flaw in this system that is often overlooked is the transportation of food. It's mindboggling. Our perpetually expanding cities and streamlined modern society seem to have discarded the common-sense concept of operating on a local level. Instead, everything is everywhere anytime all the time. And it's cheap—cheap in the sense of an over-the-counter price, but definitely not cheap in its production costs, financial and otherwise. In order for mega chain supermarkets to stock a variety of cheap goods and produce year-round, they have set up a system of transport and logistics that relies heavily on roads and trucking. Even Blind Freddy can see this system is adding to the ever-increasing problem of out of control carbon emissions. At my supermarket I can buy asparagus out of season from

Peru, apples from New Zealand, and tomatoes from Queensland in the middle of the coldest winter. Just think about the amount of gas guzzled to transport asparagus from Peru to Australia.

This system of transportation, that effectively separates us from the source of our food, has negative effects that go beyond the environmental problems it causes. Our connection to our communities and to the reality of the natural world around us also suffers. A downside of the civilized world is that we have lost the ability to depend on ourselves for essentials of everyday life. In days past our society thrived on a local economy, one that would provide for the small local community. Even in big cities, all or most of the necessary goods and services were provided locally. Times have changed and now not only have primary producers such as the market gardener disappeared but so have many of our local services, like the butchers, bakers, and fruit and vegetable shops.

Let's think for a moment about the shirt on your back. A plethora of humans all doing a small part got that shirt to you. How many people played a part in its production and ultimate delivery? The designer, the fabric maker, the seamstress, the factory manager, the department store buyer, the wholesaler, the importer, the international sailors, the warehouse staff, the delivery driver, the department store receiving dock guys, the sales staff, and finally the register operator at least, and we probably missed some. The same can be said for much of the food we consume. Now, I'm not saying that we should close down all the restaurants, cafes, and diners, far from it. I'm just saying we should all think about where our food comes from, and about the processes involved in getting that meal to our plates. Consider this hypothetical: What if the current system fell apart? It's not improbable; many successful civilizations have crumbled at their peak. How would you get your food? I know some people who can't even handle raw meat anymore, how would they survive without having someone else around to do it for them? For many the thought of killing a chicken for meat is deplorable and barbaric, but they think nothing of buying a chicken burger for lunch.

And possibly, the worst thing of all for me: all this out-of-season, long-distance-transported, mega-farmed, and overly preserved food tastes like crap!

These complex issues surrounding food production had been weighing heavily on my mind, and the more I thought about it the more frustrated I became. In fact, I was angered that I existed at this moment in time, with so many challenges for us to overcome. But despite this seemingly dire outlook, I had a determination to do something about it. I was convinced that I still had options. I still had a choice, didn't I? Surely it all came down to choice! However, the more I looked into the situation the more it appeared that I had limited choice—that is if I continued to rely on supermarkets to be my main food provider. So, I started buying my food somewhere else. I started to shop at farmer's markets. At first this seemed like a great solution, but I began to see the downsides of this as well. Our local farmer's markets began with great intentions but they now seem to be catering to a more yuppie market, offering "gourmet" prepackaged items at exuberant prices. I just want the ability to buy fresh, seasonal vegetables grown locally! Is that too much to ask? Apparently so...

Local farming exists on some level, but I discovered that in our region most of the produce gets sent to the major cities for distribution, and sometimes is then sent back to our local retailers. What a system! For example, I discovered that our local potato growers mostly supply a national chip manufacturer or send their potatoes to the city markets, but for some odd reason they don't supply our local restaurants. Even more confounding, they don't supply our local green grocery stores, which end up purchasing their produce from the city wholesale market! I wore out a patch on my noggin from constantly scratching my head, desperately trying to figure out the logic of this predicament.

I realized something had to be done; I had to take action! It was clear that I was a "food victim" and it was time to take back control. I discovered it's possible when you grow your own fruit and vegetables, raise your own meat, and know what to eat from the wild. This is how I made the switch.

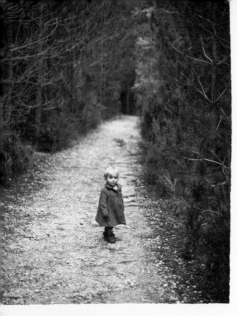
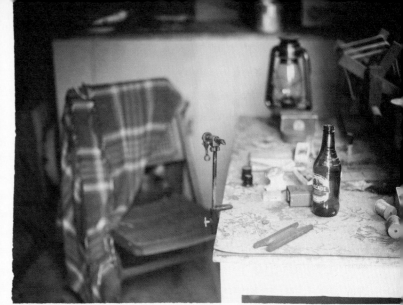
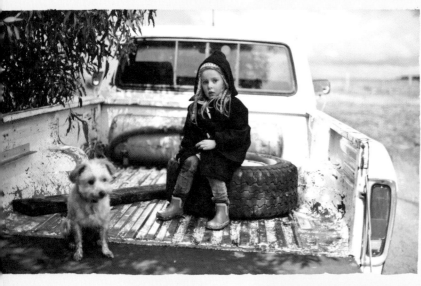
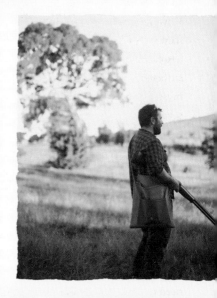
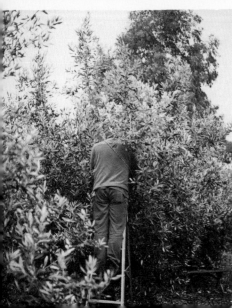
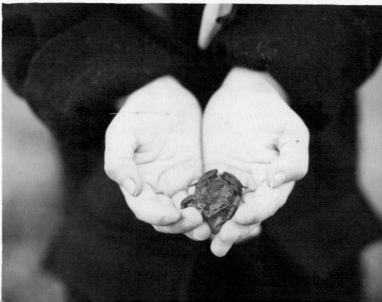

THE INITIAL STEPS

My goal was to become completely self-sufficient. I've always grown a little vegetable garden whenever I had a place with a patch of available soil. But it was never for any purpose other than just a bit of fun (yes I'm a garden nerd). Because of this, I already had most of the required skills, I had the dirt and, now, I had the motivation to get serious about vegetable production. My aim was to convert my small backyard into something edible. I had visions of fruit trees, lush vegetable patches, herb gardens, and possibly a few chooks.

Then I got the reality check: My yard was pretty small, so no chickens for us and no large orchard, either. However, there was certainly room for a handful of fruit trees espaliered along the northern-facing fence, a ton of herbs, and plenty of vegetables. Semi-self-sufficiency was becoming a real possibility. I taught myself many new tricks, like how to raise my own seedlings, which was a big money saver. I learned how to rotate crops, the intricacies of companion planting, and how to plant with less crop clustering to avoid insect predation. I learned more about the benefits of composting and the "joys" of weeding. I'm the kind of bloke who loves to learn practical skills, so the process was not a chore; it was enjoyable.

Summer has always been the peak growing season but the colder months couldn't be ignored, as we still need to have food on our plates in the winter. So I did some research and discovered viable winter crops. However, there is no way to avoid the lull in food production during the cooler months, even when you raise some winter crops, so I had to learn techniques for preserving the summer harvest.

I had the fruit and vegetables covered, but what about meat? Like most people I realize that livestock production isn't faultless. Not only does the cruelty to animals disturb me, but so do the devastating environmental effects that result from raising beef and sheep in large numbers. Poisoned water supplies, infection and disease, harmful gasses, and deforestation all result from this type of large-scale animal farming. Not to say beef and lamb production should come to a grinding halt; they taste too good. But I decided to reduce my consumption of these beasts and to be considerate of where my meat was coming from.

My solution was to look backwards, back to a time when men were men and women were women. What had my ancestors done for meat? How much meat did they eat? We already didn't eat very much red meat in our house. But I still needed to identify a reliable source of meat that would fit into my self-sustaining vision. I didn't have to look far. Meat-providing animals were everywhere and were regarded as unwanted pests. Our region is loaded with European rabbit and hare, both considered invasive and destructive species. They're fairly easy to hunt and in year-round supply. Seasonally there is also good supply of ducks, trout, eel, and yabbies (crawfish). It didn't take much research to find local farmed trout, venison, and poultry, which had the added benefit of supporting the local economy. Things were looking good for meat acquisition! Just like raising a garden, it required a bit more work than walking through the automatic doors at the supermarket, but the effort was both pleasurable and ethically and spiritually satisfying.

Our new approach to sourcing food had been covered. I also found I was able to supplement my plate with other seasonal treats that could be found growing in the wild, such as mushrooms and nettles, which required almost no effort on my part other than figuring out when and where to look for them. Now I just needed to work on the flavor factor. Luckily, this turned out to come naturally. With such fresh produce the flavor was enhanced tenfold. Until you've tasted homegrown and wild-raised food you just won't understand what I'm going on about. Not to mention the special joy you experience eating your own food. It's like you're devouring the control you've just taken back, and it's delicious.

THE WLL SYSTEM

It is important to understand that in order to get a meal onto the plate completely of your own volition, there is a good deal of behind the scenes action required. Forward thinking, seasonal planning, patience, practice, and effort are all required.

The simplest way to illustrate this is to examine the preparation of a typical dinner. Take for example a rabbit ragu to be served with pasta. Let's break down each of the elements of this meal and what is required to produce them. First, the most important element of a good ragu is passata, which is a basic tomato sauce that is made at the end of summer, bottled for use all through the year (see page 212). This requires a season of tending to tomatoes in the garden, followed by a day of work preparing and bottling the passata. Next on the list are the fresh carrots, garlic, and onions. These need to be planted at the beginning of spring for a harvest during summer and autum, and stored properly. The meat for the ragu ought to be free-range locally bought, home-raised, or hunted, the last two options each requiring a bit of planning and effort to execute. The all-important stock would preferably be made and stored frozen until required. If it's a meat stock, think about where that animal has come from. Let's not forget the fresh herbs needed. You'll need to have these growing in your yard all year round. And finally the pasta: it's one of the easiest things to make, but it takes a few more steps than just opening a cardboard box! So you can see there are multiple elements that are brought together to make the dish. Pulling this off is possible with the WLL system.

For the system to work, in addition to a functional, seasonal home garden, a larder of some sort is advised. This is where you store food items in various forms that will provide nourishment, and some flavorful variety all year round. I've seen some stunning examples online, where people have converted their laundry into a walk-in storage facility reminiscent of a nuclear fallout

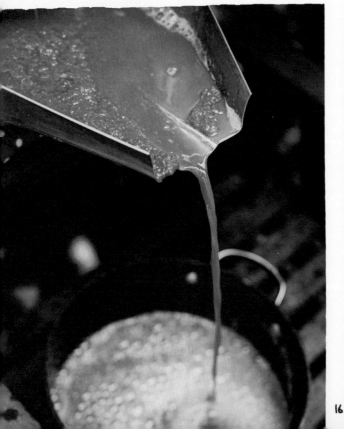

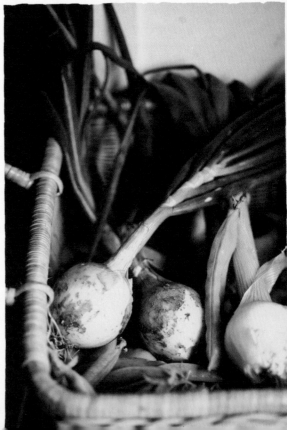

shelter. No need to go over the top. More important is what food goes inside. Make a jam or a relish from your excess garden produce, cure some pork, make sausages, hang some homegrown garlic and chili to dry. The possibilities are endless. Beans are a good example of something that grows prolifically over summer and can be dried out in their pods and harvested as dry beans, which will store indefinitely in a dry cool place—a perfect food to consume over winter. Pumpkins and potatoes, if stored properly, are also a great source of food for winter, as they keep for ages and are super versatile in the kitchen. Many of the underground vegetables like parsnip and carrots can be stored in baskets of soil and sand and will keep over winter. The more you investigate the more techniques you will find to store food. People have been doing it for thousands of years. We've just somehow lost touch with these techniques with the advent of preservatives and pre-packaged food.

Another key to the WLL system working effectively is involving your community. Share your produce with friends and family and try to create a harvest network that promotes sharing, keeping you stocked with mixed produce through the year. Harvest networks get me really excited! My friends and family are always swapping and sharing food. We've somehow managed to create a great network and I believe the more people that get involved in this sort of system the less we will rely on supermarkets—a clear win in my view. We'll always need to buy the basics like sugar, tea, coffee, salt, flour, and condoms, but it is possible to raise enough of the fresh stuff yourself to keep a family fed most of the year round. If we all did a little bit, imagine the impact we could all make.

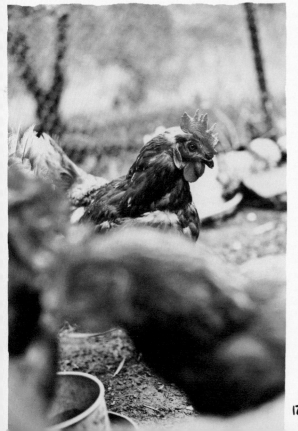

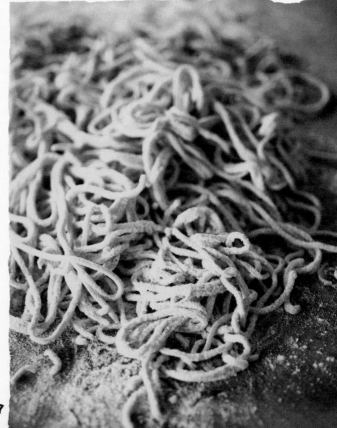

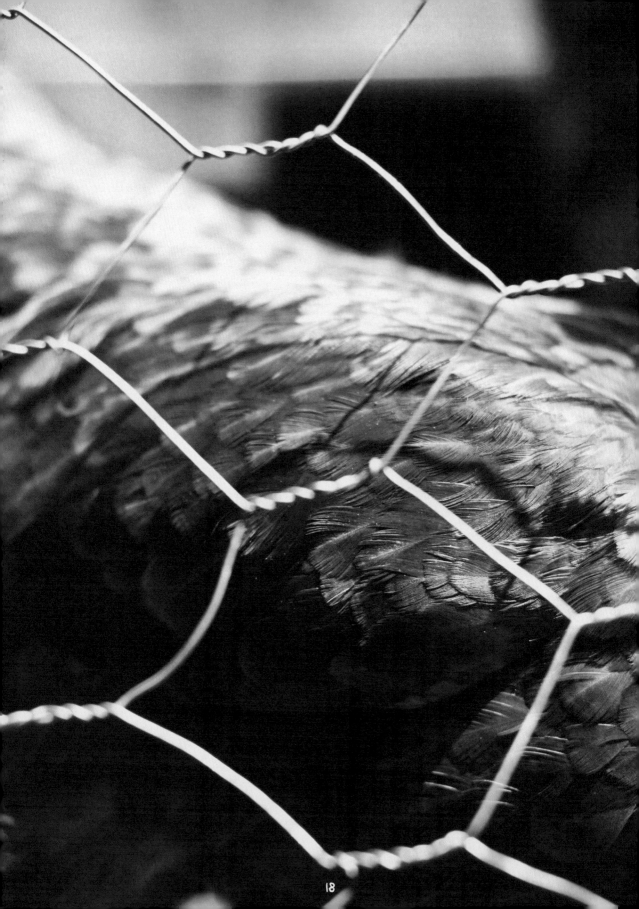

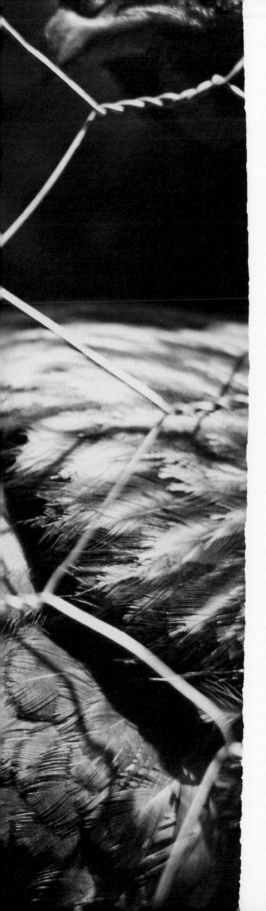

MEAT ACQUISITION

Someone once thoughtfully informed me that in this modern world we have supermarkets, where meat can be purchased with ease. I replied back, "Don't you think that's part of the problem?" Meat is a privilege, not a right. We should work hard for it, and we should be intimate with the process of taking a life to sustain our own. No matter where you live, there is always something to hunt and fish. The important things are: your motive for hunting/fishing, the amount you hunt, and how you do it. I'll make this perfectly clear. I hunt only for food not for sport. I don't hunt for trophies to hang on my wall or to feed some sick bloodlust. I hunt exclusively to put food on the plate. I don't care what anyone else does; it's their prerogative.

So, hunting is one option, and with my small yard it's the best option. However, if you have land, which is also a privilege, then there is the option of raising your own meat, such as chickens, geese, ducks, quails, pigs, and rabbits. All of these animals are relatively easy to raise, provided you have the space. You can be in control of how the animals live and eventually how they die. In the process you will find a heightened respect for your meat. Dispatching an animal is never an easy thing to do, no matter how many times you do it, so you might only do it a few times a year. My folks often remind me that, for them, eating a home raised chicken was a once or twice a year event practiced strictly on special occasions. The added benefit of raising poultry is fresh eggs. This has to be one of the greatest joys of home production. Fresh, happy eggs can turn a dull moment into a fiesta on Ibiza. Well maybe not, but they sure taste great.

Fishing is one of those funny things that men tend to do, often for all the wrong reasons. It seems to be about how big the fish is, how much money you spent on your rod, how full your tackle box is, or how many you catch. Remove all the bullshit, it should just be about the food. Again, I only fish for food. Well, actually that's a fib. I love fly-fishing because it takes me to some of the most beautiful rivers I can access. But really, I only take what I need, and once I have my quota I'm out of there.

MORE OF THE THINKING STUFF

I'm sure I've convinced you of the environmental and ethical benefits and increased quality of flavors that becoming self-sustaining will provide. However there is another, subtler, reward that we can enjoy: the innate need for a relationship with nature through the soil, plants, water, and wildlife. It's not just the final mastication of the food in the mouth, nor the joy the taste buds pass to your brain, it's bigger than that. There is a sense of satisfaction from getting your hands dirty, nurturing your food from seed, and enjoying something nature has provided, while inevitably spending time outside in the elements to make it all happen. Our basic primeval needs can be satisfied with some time spent out in the fields, foraging in the forests, and hunting and fishing as our ancestors did. Our affluent, post-industrial-revolution society looks down its nose at this rugged lifestyle, preferring the conveniences the civilized world provides. I know which I prefer.

For many of us, life is jammed with rush, noise, convenience, and stress. There is little time left for contact with the natural world. Take a minute to ask yourself about the choices you've made in life. Many people choose to live in a rushed cycle: wake up, eat a highly processed breakfast, drive to work, sit in the office, go home, eat poorly, and sit in front of the box until falling asleep, then begin the process over again the following morning. Why do we live like this? Never in our history have we been so well off, yet living such poor quality lives. Is this all there is? Surely not.

For me, nothing beats getting out among it, using all my senses to appreciate my surroundings; stripping away

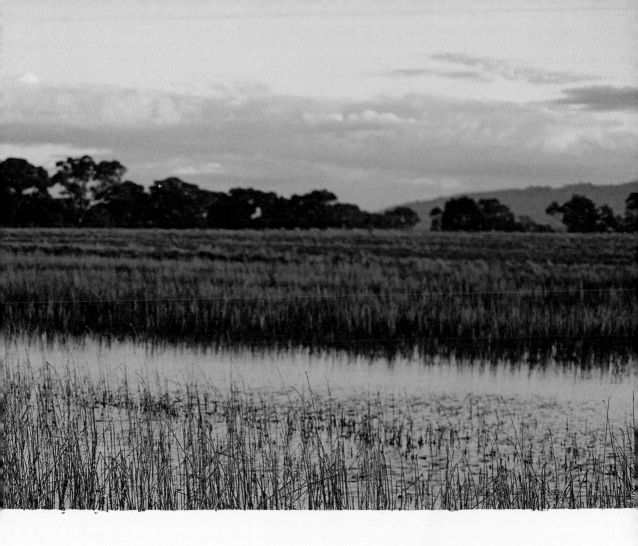

all the manmade junk to see the real world for what it is. Try spending a night out in the bush, sleeping with your back to the ground, looking up at the night sky. It's a phenomenal experience. Being immersed in nature, in the dark, allows you to hear all the night sounds: the bats, insects, birds, the breeze in the trees, and the odd mammal making its rounds. It imparts an awareness of all the other creatures and living things that we share this world with, most of which have been overlooked in our modern, synthetic world where multivitamins replace eating fresh food and enclosed gyms replace our nomadic exercise. No matter how much we try to replace our relationship with nature with manmade substitutes, we can't deny that we are in fact just links in the chain of the natural world. When all the lights turn off we will return, strangers in a strange land.

There are many cultures that live symbiotically in both worlds. I admire the lifestyles of many rural Italian communities I've visited. I saw how they utilized any available soil to grow food for the family, while raising small animals like hens, goats, and lamb. Come hunting season the men (sometimes women) would go out to catch the seasonal specialty. The produce of the forest was collected and enjoyed as a regular food source and nothing was wasted, every part of the animal was used. In these communities food is treated with respect, because they planted it, they nurtured it, they hunted it, and they ultimately ate it.

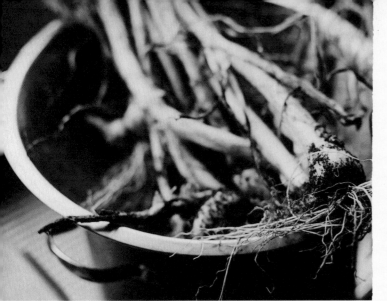

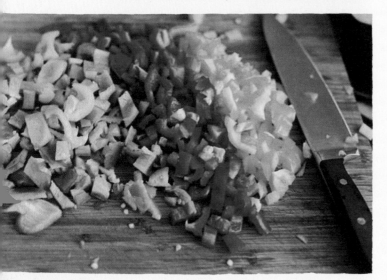

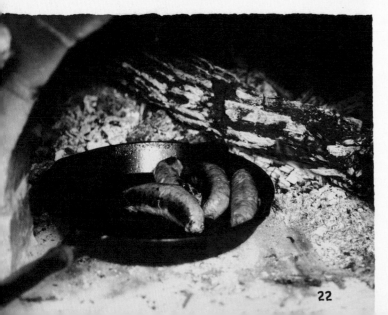

THE PEASANT COOK

This is peasant style cooking, the style I've seen Italian nonnas cook with. Nothing is strict in this book—a glug of oil, a bunch of sage, and sprinkle of salt—measurements for me are always approximate. So if I don't give a precise measurement just use what you think will work, taste it as you work, and especially before you serve it and adjust as needed. Cooking is like life; it should be free of rules, wild and free, like a naked hippy prancing in a meadow.

It should be noted that this book is full of recipes that you could cook in the weekend cabin, "log-cabineer" food one might say. It's definitely not fine food, or really fancy in any way. It's food that anyone can prepare and enjoy, from ingredients that they have raised, grown, hunted, fished, or gathered from the wild. The recipes outlined here are the ones I like to use when I'm hungry, and I hope you will enjoy them too!

All the meals in this book I cook with my backyard produce, animals that we've raised or are given to us, or food I've hunted, fished, or foraged for. If you don't have this option, then try to buy local as much as possible. This approach to food should by no means prevent you from venturing out for dinner, ordering takeout sushi, or devouring a burger. It's simply about balance. Eat more of the things you produce less of the things you don't. Ask where your food comes from—don't be shy. If you have space, then I urge you to grow, and grow like crazy. I bet you will enjoy the food and lifestyle so much that you'll wonder why you haven't always lived this way!

Welcome to Whole Larder Love...

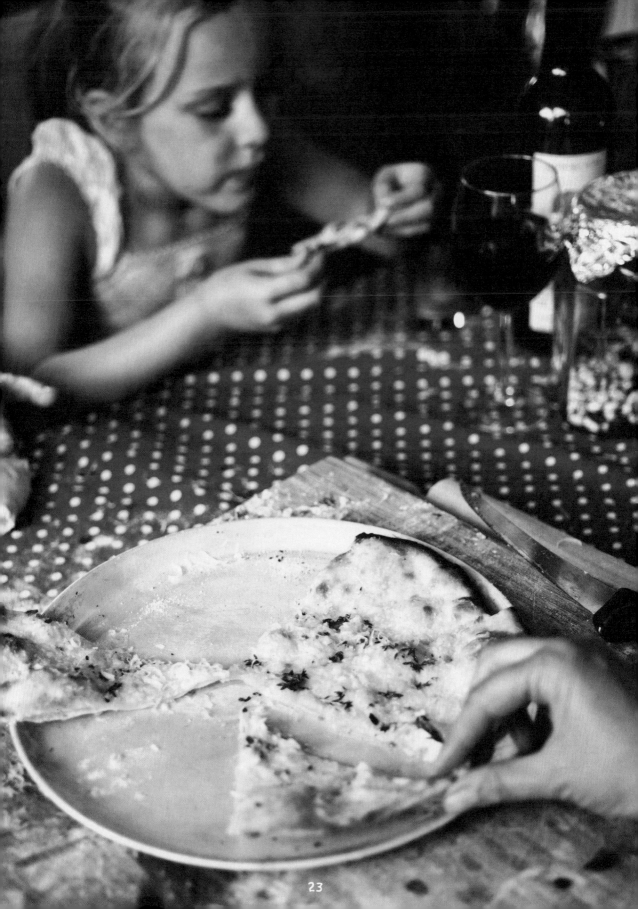

FROM TH

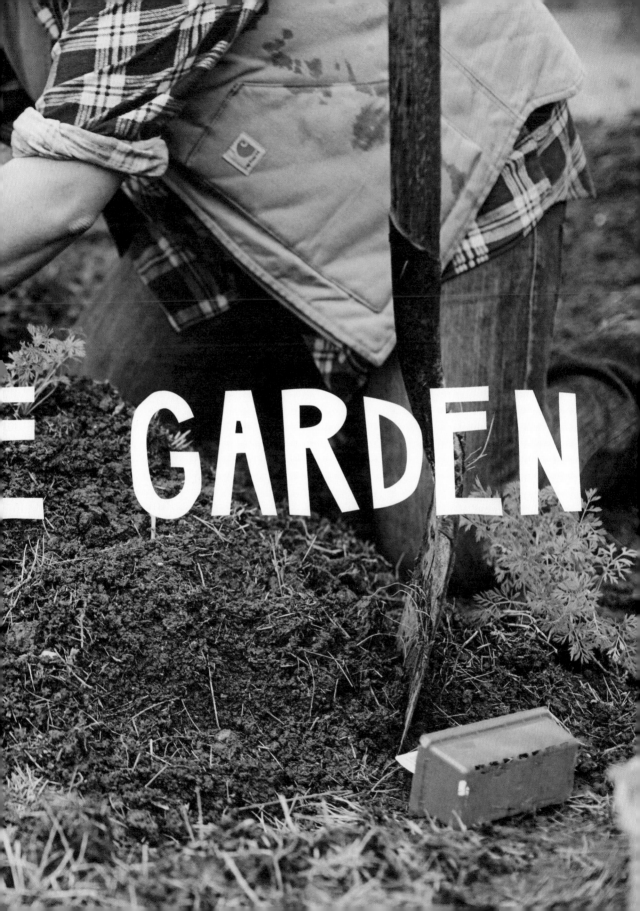

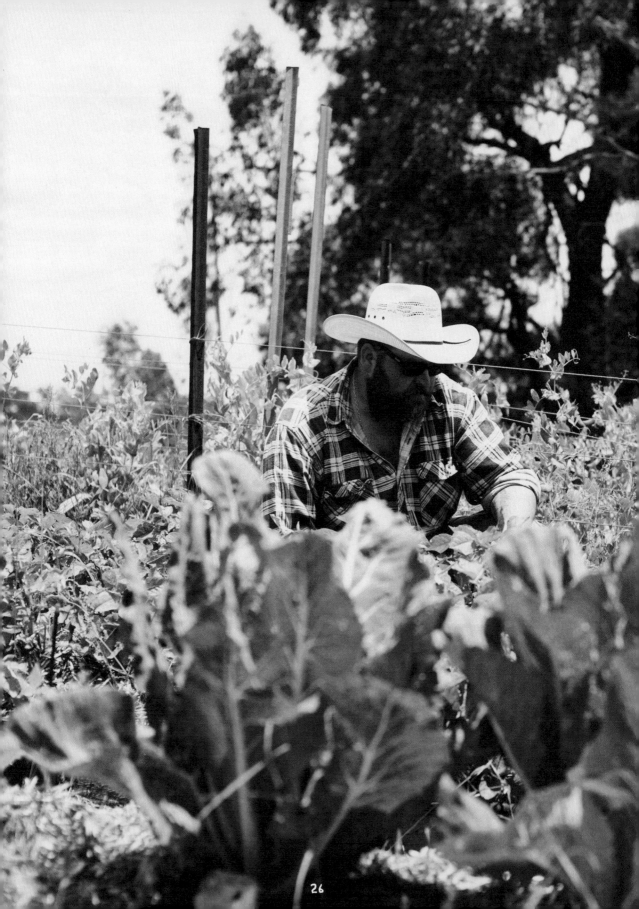

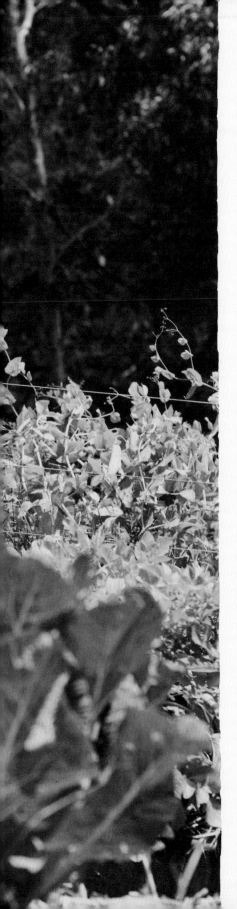

I view the garden in seasons. Tomato, zucchini, borlotti beans, and squash immediately make me think of hot summer nights puttering in the garden with a cold beer reward just around the corner. They're the kind of summer vegetables that provide me with speedy, "watch-and-grow" development. Kale, spinach, broad beans, and sprouting broccoli get me thinking of winter, when everything slows right down and anything fresh is very welcome.

Despite what most people think, maintaining a little veg patch is not hard work. The idea is to keep it simple. Start with only one or two vegetables in your first season, then build up the range from there. This approach allows you to pay more attention to your plants initially without becoming bewildered by too much too soon. These few plants will get plenty of attention, just like a new romance, and will reward you with a good harvest of fruit. The following year you'll be gagging to set up a bigger crop.

The taste of the first tomato of the new season is best described as either spiritual or orgasmic. One of my most anticipated moments of the year is the first tomato on toast with olive oil, salt, and pepper. Shudder. Tomatoes are an excellent proving ground for any budding gardener; they're pretty hardy and produce the most amazing variation of flavors. They also grow well in pots, and if you use a decent potting mix and keep the water up in summer they make an excellent option for apartment balconies or rooftops.

Growing your own tomatoes is only the tip of the iceberg. There are so many varieties of fruit, vegetables, mushrooms, nuts, and olives that you can grow. It's a journey in itself learning what to grow and how to grow it. Keep in mind that it's best to only plant food you normally eat to begin with and avoid the urge to go crazy planting a heap of exotic vegetables you don't normally cook with. Leave them for the future when you want something different.

If you are shy of growing veggies, and very limited for space, then try a little herb garden of the tough stuff like rosemary, thyme, and oregano. Just pop them in a pot, keep the moisture up, and then be amazed by the intensity they will bring to your cooking. If you don't already use fresh herbs then the change will blow you away. There is a great sense of satisfaction in growing your own, and it's definitely worth the small effort required to set it up.

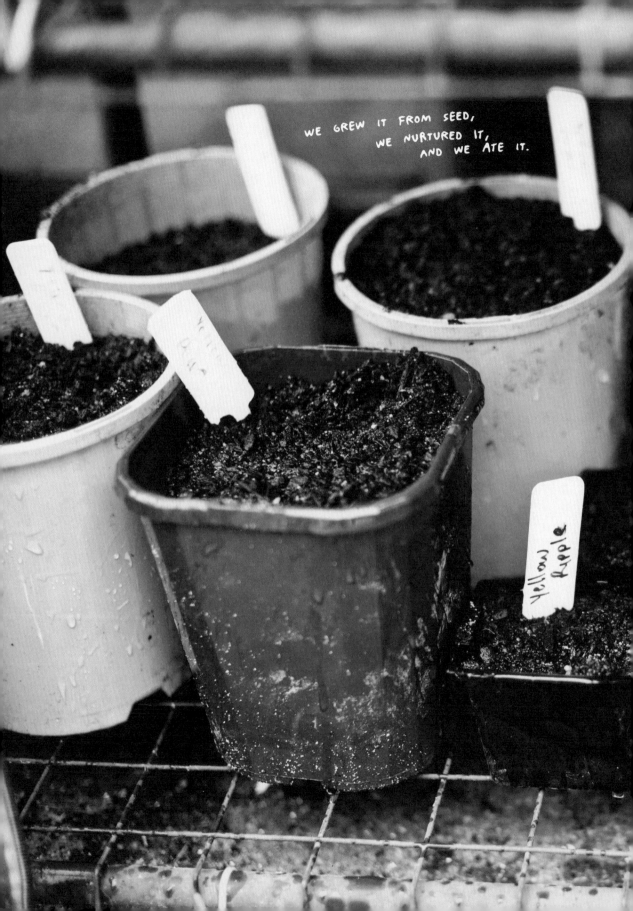

WE GREW IT FROM SEED,
WE NURTURED IT,
AND WE ATE IT.

EXACTLY WHAT MY MUM TAUGHT ME
ALL THOSE YEARS AGO ON THE FARM.

Yellow Ripple

Yellow Ripple

Yellow Ripple

CHEERS TO YOU, MUM.

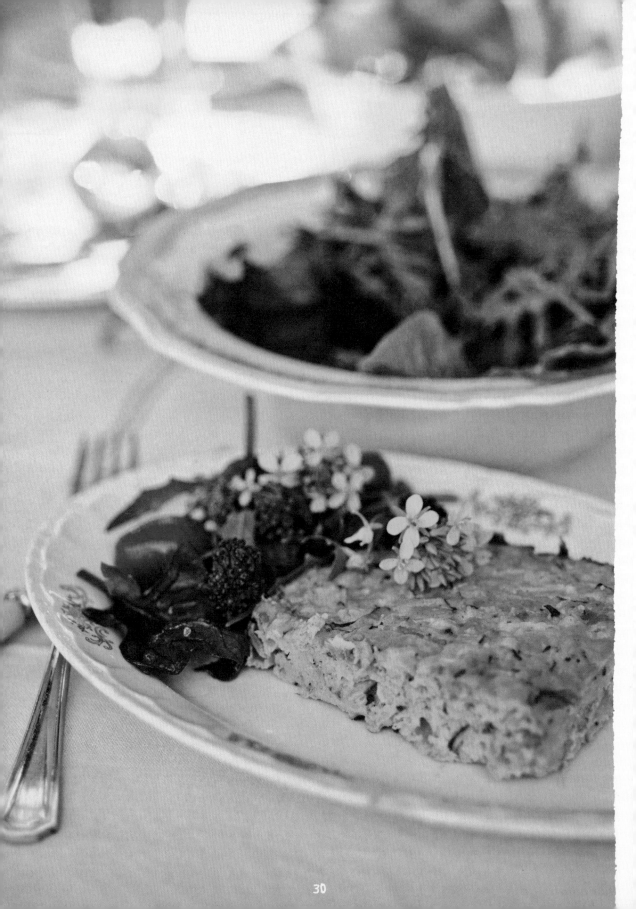

SLICE OF SPRING

I REALLY LIKE MEALS THAT ARE SIMPLE TO MAKE, THE ONES THAT ARE PERFECTLY SUITED FOR WEEKNIGHT DINNERS WHEN THERE ALWAYS SEEM TO BE OTHER DISTRACTIONS AROUND. AND TO BE HONEST, WE ALL GET A LITTLE LAZY, SO ANYTHING SIMPLE CAN BE VERY APPEALING. THIS MEAL MAKES THE MOST OF YOUR FRESH EGGS AND THE PROLIFIC VEGGIES ZUCCHINI AND SPINACH. YOU CAN SERVE IT COLD OR HOT, AND WHEN THE ZUCCHINI IS IN SEASON IT MAKES A GREAT SPRING MEAL WITH A FRESH SALAD OF ALL YOUR GARDEN LEAVES AND FLOWERS.

WHAT YOU NEED:

6 x eggs
7 oz (200 g) rindless bacon, chopped
2 x medium zucchini, grated
Handful of baby spinach, finely chopped
1 x large onion, finely chopped
1 cup self-raising flour
1 cup grated Parmesan
1 cup grated cheddar cheese
1 tsp cumin
1 tsp garam masala
1 tsp curry powder
Ground sea salt
Ground black pepper
Glug of olive oil
Butter

HOW TO:

Preheat the oven to 340 F (170 C).

Grease an approximately 8 x 12 in (20 x 30 cm) baking dish with butter.

Beat the eggs in a large bowl.

Stir in the zucchini, spinach, bacon, flour, cheddar and Parmesan cheese, onion, and oil. Then add spices and season to taste with salt and pepper.

Pour mixture into the greased dish and bake uncovered for 30 minutes.

Grate over some extra Parmesan and serve with a fresh garden salad.

ZUCCHINI GARGANELLI

MOST OF US HAVE MEALS THAT OUR MUMS COOKED THAT HAVE BECOME A STAPLE SOURCE OF COMFORT FOOD. FOR AS LONG AS I CAN REMEMBER, MUM HAS COOKED A CREAMY, ZUCCHINI AND BACON PASTA THAT OUR WHOLE FAMILY LOVES. IT'S A MEAL THAT (SURPRISE, SURPRISE) AROSE FROM HER NEED TO USE UP EXCESS ZUCCHINI FROM HER GARDEN! IT WAS SUCH A SIMPLE MEAL THAT IT WAS OFTEN COOKED ON BUSY WEEKNIGHTS. I'VE CONTINUED TO COOK IT, WITH JUST A FEW TWEAKS, MAINLY REPLACING THE BACON WITH OUR HOME-CURED PROSCIUTTO.

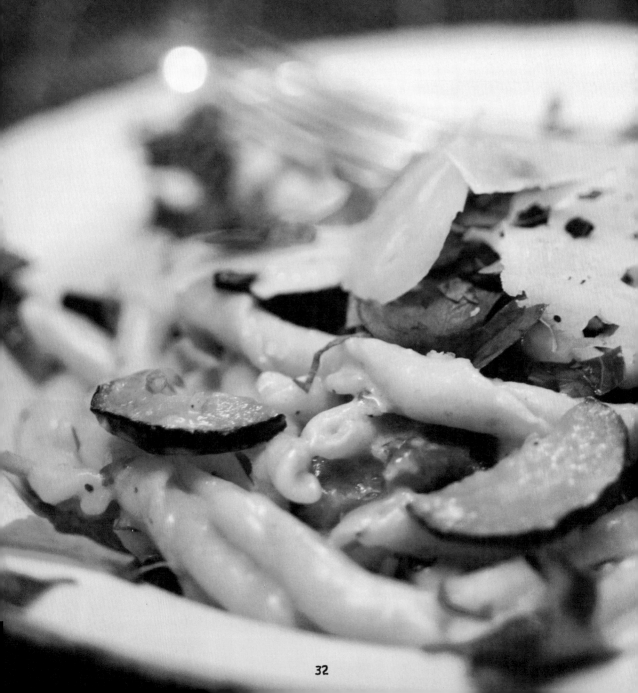

BUT IF YOU DON'T CURE YOUR OWN MEAT, THEN YOU CAN USE BACON OR STORE-BOUGHT PROSCIUTTO. THIS IS A FOOD TAKEN STRAIGHT FROM THE "GOOD LIFE" BIBLE, WITH MOST OF THE INGREDIENTS POTENTIALLY COMING STRAIGHT FROM YOUR BACKYARD OR LARDER. IF YOU GROW YOUR OWN ZUCCHINI TRY THE YELLOW AND BLACK TYPES TO MIX UP THE COLOR ON THE PLATE SOMEWHAT.

WHAT YOU NEED:

6 slices prosciutto, stripped

1 lb (500 g) garganelli pasta

2 x medium zucchini, sliced

10 x ripe cherry tomato, halved

4 x cloves garlic, chopped

1/2 cup Parmesan cheese

1/2 cup (125 ml) pouring cream

1 handful fresh parsley, chopped

Olive oil

Salt

Pepper

HOW TO:

Slice the zucchini any way you want. I normally slice it down the center, then into smaller, bite-size chunks.

Boil a large pot of salted water and start cooking the garganelli.

Heat a glug of oil in a frying pan.

Panfry the zucchini for five minutes and then add the prosciutto and cook for another five minutes. The zucchini should be nicely browned and the prosciutto getting crisp.

Now add the garlic, tomatoes, and parsley (leaving some for garnish). Stir well.

Reduce the heat to a low simmer.

When the garganelli is al dente, strain and return it to the pot it was cooked in.

Pour in the sauce, add the cream and Parmesan, and season and stir well.

Garnish with the remaining parsley, grate some fresh Parmesan on top, and dress with olive oil.

Serve with ciabatta bread and a fine Pinot Noir.

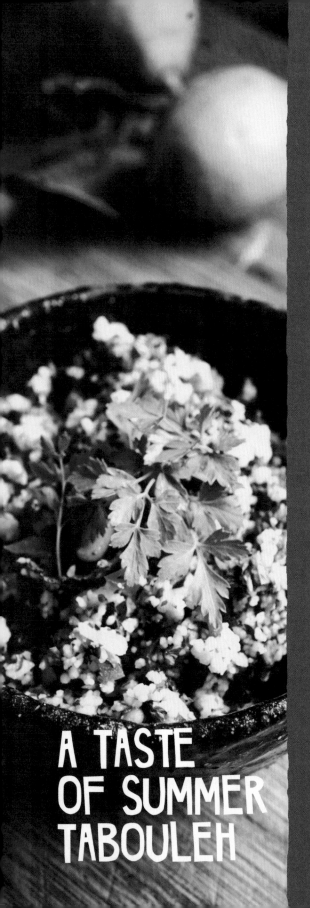

During the warmer months this salad gets a hammering at our place. I just love the fact that I can walk out to the yard, pick a bunch of parsley, mint, grab a lemon, pluck a few tomatoes, and pull out a small onion, and voilà! It's summer in a nutshell! picked and placed in my basket, ready to make a fresh salad.

Originating in Lebanon, this salad is traditionally held together using bulgur wheat, which is easy to cook, but sometimes difficult to find. So, if you can't get access to bulgur, then couscous is an alternative. It should be noted that traditionally more parsley than mint is used, with parsley dominating flavor-wise, but play around with it to suit your tastes. Also of note is that a traditional tabouleh will have more parsley than bulgur or couscous but we're not in Lebanon so make it how you like it.

What you need:

1 cup couscous
1 x small onion, diced
3 x tomatoes, finely chopped
2 x lemons, juice
1 cup parsley, finely chopped
1/2 cup mint, finely chopped
1 handful pine nuts
1/4 cup olive oil
Salt
Pepper

How to:

Prepare the couscous as per packet instructions. When done, allow to cool.

Heat a glug of olive oil in a frying pan, and panfry the pine nuts until they brown. Around 5 minutes will do. You just want to get some color into them, not burn them. When they're done, remove from heat and allow them to cool (just a few minutes).

In a large mixing bowl mix all the ingredients well.

Taste the salad, add the juice of another lemon if needed, and season.

Easy!

A TASTE OF SUMMER TABOULEH

SUMMER BRUSCHETTA

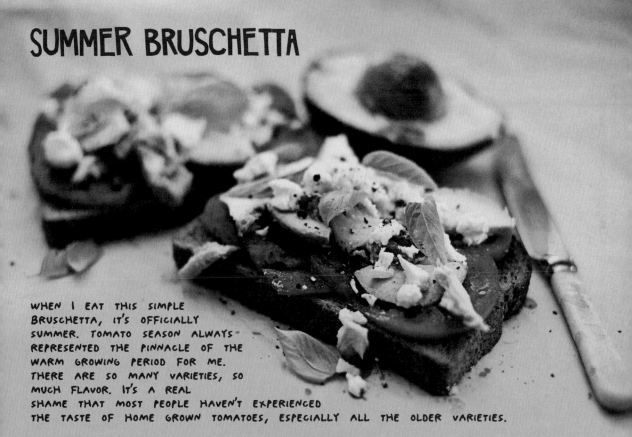

WHEN I EAT THIS SIMPLE BRUSCHETTA, IT'S OFFICIALLY SUMMER. TOMATO SEASON ALWAYS REPRESENTED THE PINNACLE OF THE WARM GROWING PERIOD FOR ME. THERE ARE SO MANY VARIETIES, SO MUCH FLAVOR. IT'S A REAL SHAME THAT MOST PEOPLE HAVEN'T EXPERIENCED THE TASTE OF HOME GROWN TOMATOES, ESPECIALLY ALL THE OLDER VARIETIES.

IT'S TAKEN ME A FEW YEARS TO FIND THE VARIETIES THAT ARE BEST SUITED TO OUR CLIMATE, ONE OF THEM BEING ROUGE DE MARMANDE. EVER HEARD OF IT? WELL NEITHER HAD I UNTIL ABOUT FIVE YEARS AGO WHEN A LOCAL POLISH GROWER INTRODUCED ME TO IT. HE SAID IT WAS THE BEST CROPPER AND FLAVOR PROVIDER IN HIS HUMBLE OPINION. IT'S BEEN ONE OF MY FAVORITE VARIETIES EVER SINCE. IF YOU'RE THINKING OF GROWING YOUR OWN TOMATOES I URGE YOU TO TRY. EVEN IF IT'S IN A POT ON AN APARTMENT BALCONY IN THE CITY, OR IN A SUBURBAN YARD, THE EXPERIENCE WILL ENRICH YOUR SUMMER DAYS.

IF YOU CAN SOURCE MEREDITH DAIRY MARINATED GOATS CHEESE FROM YOUR DELI, GRAB IT. IT'S DIVINE. IF NOT, THERE ARE PLENTY OF OPTIONS FOR GOAT'S FETA.

WHAT YOU NEED:

Ciabatta bread, sliced
Mixed tomatoes, mixed colors
Ripe avocado
1 x clove garlic
Meredith Dairy Marinated
  Goats Cheese
Parmesan cheese
Basil
Olive oil
Salt
Pepper

HOW TO:

Slice the tomatoes and set aside in a bowl. Sprinkle with a little salt.

Toast the sliced ciabatta. When it's toasted and hot, rub the sliced garlic clove over each side.

Place the tomato on the bread, and place the goat's feta and a few slices of avocado on top.

Grate over some Parmesan, dress with olive oil, and garnish with some fresh basil leaves.

Season with cracked S&P.

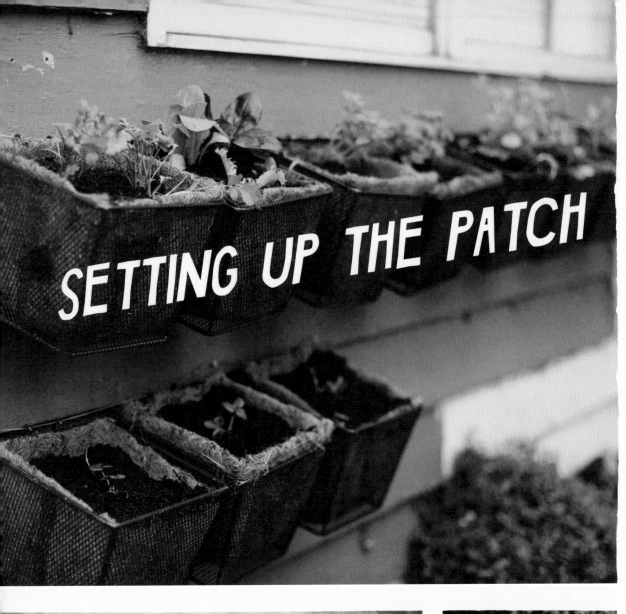

SETTING UP THE PATCH

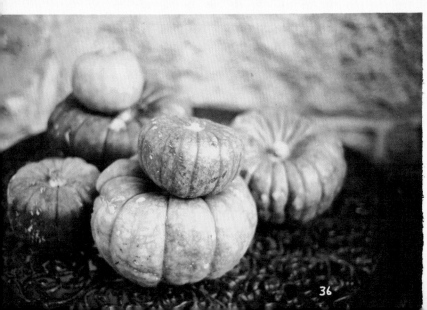

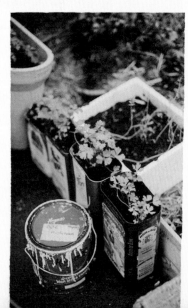

Most likely we all had a go at growing seedlings back in primary school. If not, don't be alarmed. I like to dispense with rules and instead learn by trial and error. Just keep in mind the basics: soil, seed, sun, and water. Seriously it's that easy. You put a seed in the soil where it will get sunlight, water it, and admire as nature goes to work.

Raising your own seedlings is a good way to save a bunch of money. A little bit of effort can go a long way. In early spring, mid-spring, and mid-summer, I'll set aside some time to propagate all of my seedlings. I use a very simple and efficient method: the toilet roll system. During the year I save all those toilet rolls that would otherwise be discarded and end up in a landfill. When they are filled with a seed raising mix (available at your local nursery) they make a great home for young seedlings. It's simply a matter of popping in the seed (read the packet for instructions) and keeping the sunlight and moisture up. In a few weeks, out come the seedlings; a few weeks of development later and the plant and its toilet roll home can be planted straight into the garden, with no damage to the delicate root system. The paper roll will eventually rot away. It's a proven method that I urge you to try.

If you have a backyard with plenty of space and it's currently filled with ornamentals and grass, pick a sunny spot and start a little plot. You don't have to tear down the rest of your garden and make a mini farmlet. Our garden space is very modest and quite small, so it's all edible plants, and as far as aesthetics go I couldn't think of anything prettier. You may want to enlarge your setup after a few seasons, but start small to begin with, plant the vegetables and herbs that you use regularly and plant them in small batches.

For those living in apartments, if you have a balcony or access to the rooftop then you're blessed. You can grow a heap in pots, especially in the summer. Just make sure they get the basic necessities, especially water. Imagine your own fresh tomatoes, lettuce, and basil; again it's just a matter of soil, seed, sunlight, and water. I have plenty of friends that grow a good deal in very tight spaces. Many of them grow the type of things that are used in small batches in the kitchen such as lettuce, tomato, celery, carrots, eggplant, zucchini, and all the herbs they need. It's just a matter of going out to the balcony picking a few basil leaves, a tomato or two, and you have the fresh makings of a summer bruschetta.

The key to a profitable and functional vegetable patch is planning. Take a moment to think about what you like to eat, and then learn how long that particular vegetable will take to mature. There is no point having the literal fruits of your labor rotting on the vine because you planted too much all at once, so with that in mind be sure to also stagger your plantings over the growing season; e.g. plant a few zucchini in spring and some in mid-summer.

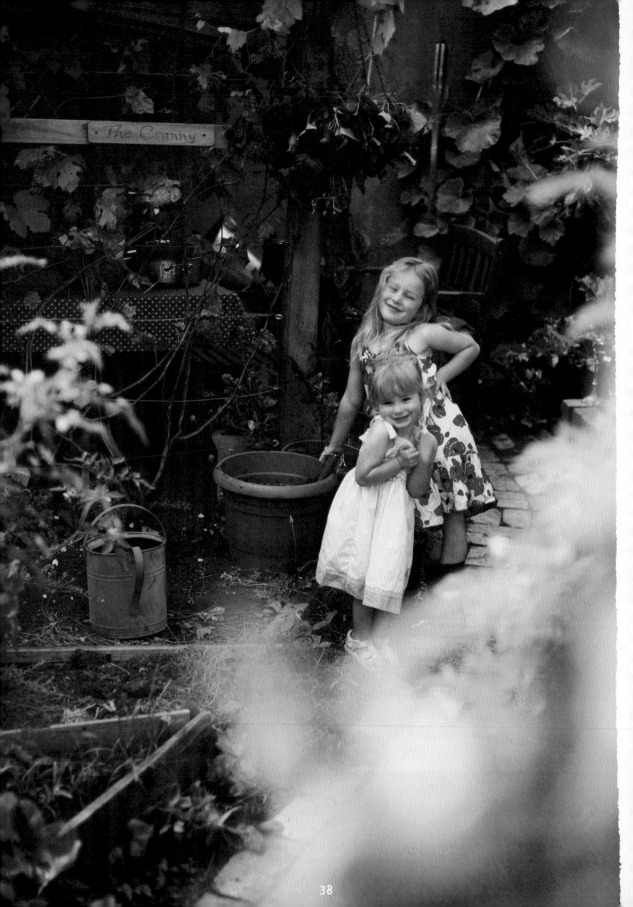

THIS IS THE SIMPLEST OF PLEASURES. IT'S SO SIMPLE IT REALLY DOESN'T EVEN NEED TO BE IN A COOKBOOK, BUT I PROMISED MY KIDS THAT THEIR FAVORITE PANCAKE TOPPING WOULD END UP IN THE BOOK. FIRST, YOU'LL NEED TO GROW THE BLUEBERRIES, OR DO A SPOT OF URBAN FORAGING AND PICK THEM FROM PLANTS WHERE THEY WOULD NORMALLY FALL TO THE GROUND. CAN YOU BELIEVE THAT ACTUALLY HAPPENS? WHAT A WASTE! AND BY TAKING THEM FROM SOMEONE ELSE'S PLANT THEY ACTUALLY TASTE BETTER. GO FIGURE. IF YOU'RE A KILLJOY, THEN YOU CAN BUY THEM, BUT IT REALLY DEFEATS THE PURPOSE OF GETTING THE BEST OF THAT FRESH, JUST-PICKED-FROM-THE-BUSH TASTE.

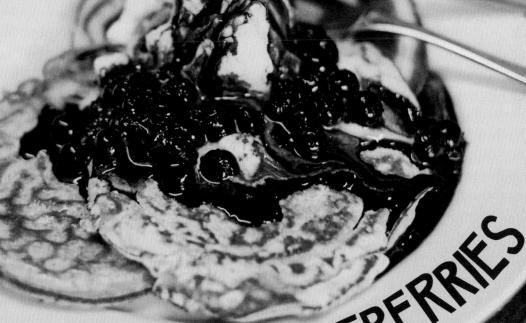

GLAZED BLUEBERRIES

WHAT YOU NEED:

7 oz (200 g) blueberries
1 tbsp white sugar
Pinch of cinnamon (optional)

HOW TO:

Heat a small saucepan, add the blueberries, the sugar, and if you're keen, the cinnamon.

Stir a little so the sugar coats the berries.

After 5 minutes the berries will be hot, the sugar and the juice will have combined to make it saucy. Pour over pancakes.

Watch children devour, looking at you like you're some sort of food magician.

LESSON TO BE LEARNT FROM TODAY:

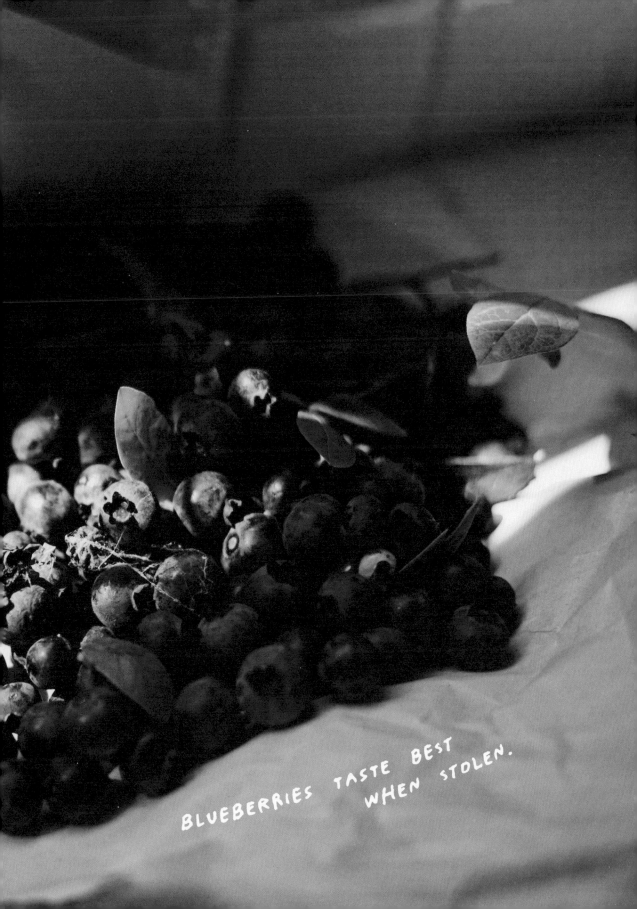

BLUEBERRIES TASTE BEST WHEN STOLEN.

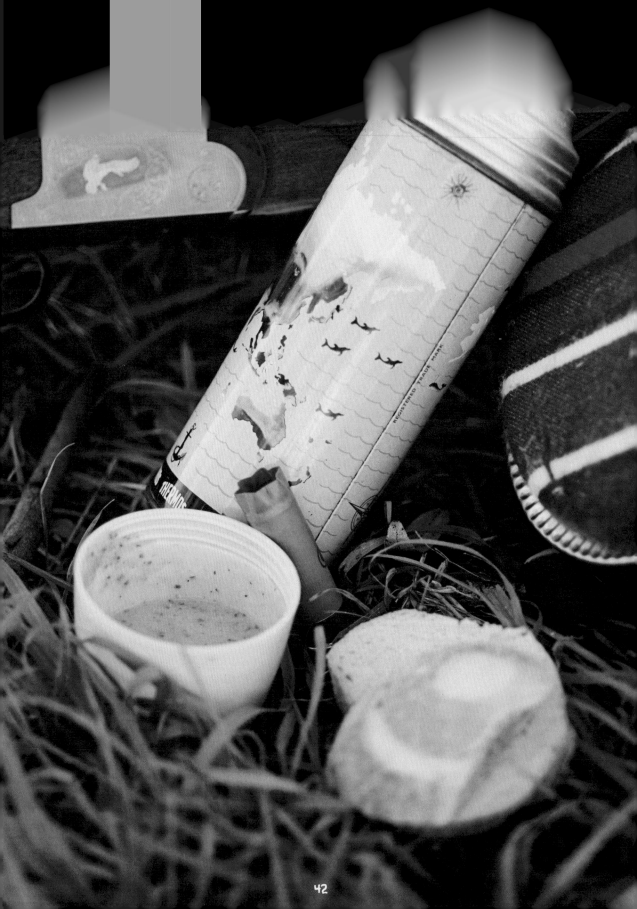

AUNTY'S ZUCCHINI SOUP

At the end of one successful summer I had a glut of zucchini and our friend (fondly referred to by our kids as Aunty) gave me this recipe to use up my unending amount of fresh, home-grown zucchini. I still haven't learned to plant the right amount of zucchini; actually I don't think anyone who has grown zucchini has ever planted the right amount. I'll often have so much that I can't give it all away, and late in the season some always feeds hordes of hungry slugs and mice. This is why I recommend growing zucchini to people just starting their own vegetable gardens—because it's super easy to grow and a ridiculously prolific producer.

You can make this soup minus the meat, and miraculously it will become a vegetarian meal! I however like the edge the prosciutto provides. It just gives it that little bit of rock and roll, reminiscent of a drug-infused Stones album.

WHAT YOU NEED:

5.25 oz (150 g) prosciutto, chopped

3 x large zucchini, roughly chopped

1 x large onion, chopped

5 x cloves garlic, chopped

2 tablespoons light sour cream

2 cups chicken stock

2 cups of water

Parmesan cheese

Olive oil

Salt

Pepper

HOW TO:

Heat oil in a saucepan. Cook the chopped prosciutto until golden brown. Set aside.

In the same saucepan heat olive oil and brown the zucchini, onion, and garlic until soft. Give it well over 5 minutes.

Add stock and water, and browned prosciutto. Season with salt and pepper.

Cook on medium heat for 15 minutes, it should reduce slightly.

Blend with a stick blender.

Serve with a good grating of quality Parmesan and some crusty bread.

THERE ARE MANY TYPES OF PUMPKIN YOU CAN GROW, AND THESE DAYS THERE IS A GREAT RANGE OF HEIRLOOM VARIETIES BECOMING MORE READILY AVAILABLE. OFTEN THOUGH, I CAN'T HELP BUT RAISE ONE OF MY OLD RELIABLE FAVORITES; THE GOOD OLD BUTTERNUT PUMPKIN (BUTTERNUT SQUASH). YOU'LL BE ABLE TO FIND SEEDLINGS AT YOUR LOCAL NURSERY OR YOU CAN PROPAGATE THEM FROM SEED USING THE TOILET ROLL METHOD (PAGE 37).

WHY IS BUTTERNUT PUMPKIN SO SPECIAL? IT'S SWEET AND NUTTY, ROASTS WELL, AND WORKS AMAZINGLY WELL IN A SOUP WHERE OTHERS FAIL TO RATE. BEST OF ALL IF YOU LEAVE AT LEAST 6 IN (15 CM) OF STALK ATTACHED WHEN YOU HARVEST THEM, THEY CAN BE STORED IN THE LARDER AND AVAILABLE FOR WINTER CONSUMPTION.

BUTTERNUT + LEEK SOUP

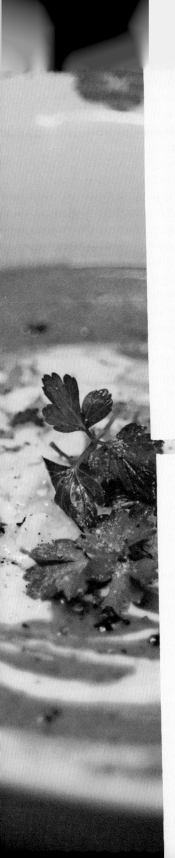

WHAT YOU NEED:

1 x butternut pumpkin, skinned
   and de-seeded
2 x leeks, chopped
5 x cloves garlic, chopped
1/2 cup grated Grana Padano
   cheese
2 tbsp butter
1/5 cup (50ml) pouring cream
1 quart (1 liter) chicken stock
Handful fresh thyme, chopped
Small handful parsley, chopped
1/2 tsp nutmeg, grated
   (or ground nutmeg)
Extra virgin olive oil
Salt
Pepper

HOW TO:

Preheat the oven to 425 F (220 C).

Clean out pumpkin and chop into
large chunks.

Place pumpkin pieces into a
roasting tray with a good drizzle of
olive oil. Get your hands right in
there and toss them around so the
pumpkin is nicely covered in that
beautiful olive oil.

Pop in your garlic cloves for
roasting too, not chopped, just
whole cloves, skin on.

Roast the pumpkin for 40
minutes turning once. When done
remove the pumpkins and garlic
and set aside.

Now heat a large saucepan,
add a glug of olive oil and the
butter. When the butter is almost
melted add the chopped leek
and cook until it softens on a
medium-high heat (normally
5-10 minutes).

Now, add the roasted pumpkin,
grate in the nutmeg, and add the
thyme and stock.

Squeeze out that wonderful soft
garlic right into your saucepan.
Try not to eat it straight away like
I always do!

Mash it all together. Use whatever
you have around; I'll often
use a potato masher or a large
wooden spoon. Don't worry
about consistency or texture at
this stage, as we'll run a whizzer
through it soon.

This is your soup base. Bring to a
boil then simmer for 15 minutes,
with a little stirring every so
often. If it looks too thick, add
more stock or hot water and stir
through.

Run a hand food processor (or a
stick blender) through the soup
to get your desired consistency.
Add your cheese, salt and pepper
to season, and stir through.

Pour in the cream, garnish with
the chopped parsley. Serve with
some toasted bread and eat away
your winter blues.

NUTS ABOUT FRUIT

There are so many small trees, dwarf varieties, bushes, and creepers such as citrus, berries, and bay, which can be grown in pots, making them a viable option for small yards and balconies. However, if you have plenty of space, there is nothing as pretty as rows of berries, fruit, and nut trees in bloom in the early weeks of spring. Not only do they look amazing but they provide the added bonus of a summer harvest of fruit and nuts which are free of chemicals and available to eat straight off the branch. Most fruit you buy at a supermarket has been picked unripe and then finishes the ripening process in transport and storage, resulting in a taste very different from fruit picked ripe off the tree. You'll often hear people going on about the how the taste of fruit and vegetables picked and eaten fresh is wildly different than store-bought varieties. Allowing fruit to ripen naturally rewards you with a completely different taste, because the natural sugars are able to develop and do their job—which in biological terms is to convince you to eat it! In turn, you go forth and deposit their seeds thus securing their genetic signature. Science is rad!

Like I mentioned earlier, I have space restrictions in my yard, but somehow I've managed to fit a selection of fruit, nuts, and citrus in my modest space. The trick is to train the tree to grow flat along a wall; this, in gardening terms, is to "espalier." Each year as the new wood grows you tie the young branches to something flat against a wall, fence, or building. All trees naturally grow upwards, so it's just a matter of training them to grow sideways instead, which will make the most of a small space. It's not an art form, just common sense. And they fruit the same as when left to their own devices.

Fruit trees may need a pruning in winter. This sometimes can be intimidating, as it can be hard to determine what to cut back, and nobody wants to cut too much. There are no hard and fast rules, just trim to the bud. Again, you will learn this skill after a few seasons.

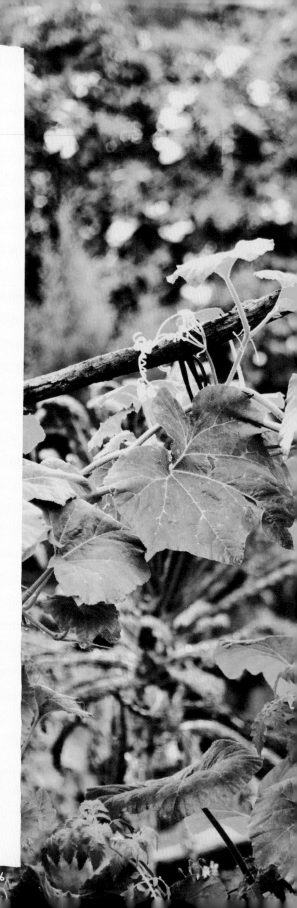

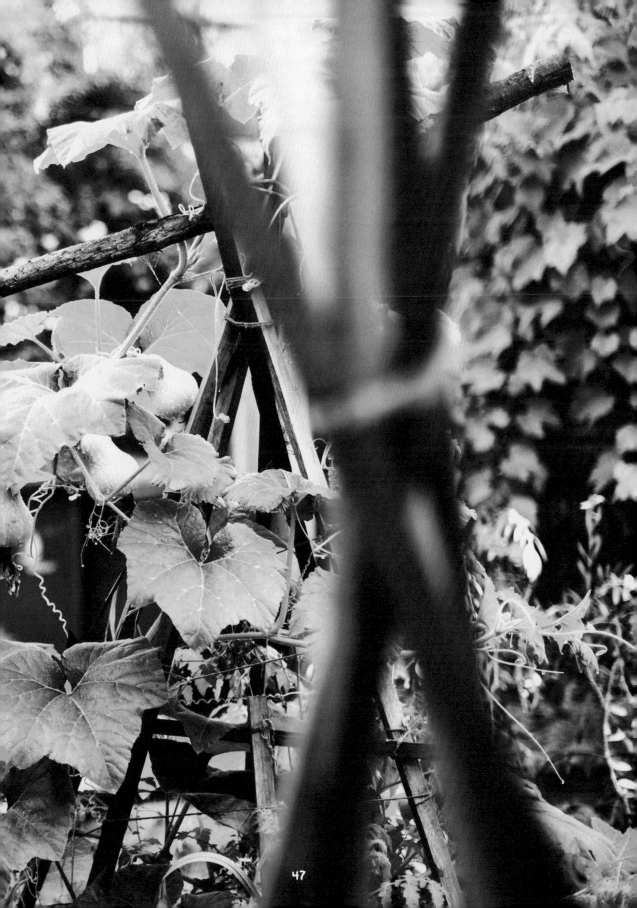

POTIMARRON + GORGONZOLA SOUP

I PLACE PUMPKIN IN THE SAME CATEGORY AS ZUCCHINI REGARDING EASE OF GROWING. EVEN IF YOU DON'T HAVE MUCH SPACE IN YOUR YARD, PUMPKINS CAN BE TRAINED TO GROW UP ALMOST ANYTHING RESEMBLING A TRELLIS. I HAVE THIS VISION OF TRAINING A PUMPKIN USING THE OLD CIRCUS METHOD WITH A CHAIR, A WHIP, AND A PITH HELMET (BUT THIS APPROACH IS TOTALLY UNNECESSARY, USE GARDEN TIES INSTEAD). AS THE PLANT GROWS, TIE IT TO SOMETHING LIKE A FENCE OR TRELLIS AND FORCE IT TO GROW UP INSTEAD OF OUTWARDS. IF YOU PREFER THE WHIP AND CHAIR METHOD BY ALL MEANS GO AHEAD, I WON'T JUDGE YOU. I MADE A TRELLIS OUT OF PINE WILDLINGS THAT I THATCHED TOGETHER TO MAKE A SORT OF ROUGH GRID, AND WITH EACH NEW GROWTH I'D TIE IT AND WATCHED IT REACH STUNNING HEIGHTS OF ALMOST NINE FEET! THE BEAUTY OF THIS SYSTEM IS THAT YOU ARE MAKING USE OF A SPACE THAT WAS OTHERWISE UNPRODUCTIVE.

THE FRENCH PUMPKIN VARIETY POTIMARRON IS ONE OF MY FAVORITES TO CULTIVATE. IT'S A BEAUTIFUL ALL-ROUNDER, AND MY PREFERRED PUMPKIN TO GROW EACH SEASON, OTHER THAN THE BUTTERNUT. IF YOU HAVEN'T TRIED IT BEFORE I RECOMMEND JUST EATING IT ROASTED INITIALLY, TO EXPERIENCE ITS UNIQUE FLAVOR. IF YOU CAN'T GET YOUR HANDS ON SEEDLINGS OR BUY THEM AT YOUR MARKET, THEN SUBSTITUTE IT WITH A BUTTERNUT PUMPKIN. I NORMALLY BUY MY SEEDS FOR THIS OLD VARIETY ONLINE.

WHAT YOU NEED:

Ciabatta bread, sliced

1 x whole potimarron pumpkin, peeled and chopped into chunks

1 x onion, chopped

5 x cloves garlic, chopped

5.25 oz (150 g) Gorgonzola cheese

1 cup thickened cream

3.5 oz (100 g) pine nuts

1 quart (1 liter) chicken stock

Sprig of fresh parsley, chopped

1 tsp cumin seeds

1 tsp garam masala

1 tsp dried thyme, chopped

2 tsp curry powder

Pepper

Salt

HOW TO:

Preheat the oven to 400 F (200 C).

Place peeled pumpkin chunks into roasting dish, cover with a glug of olive oil and mix well. Roast until soft on the inside. Test one to see if it's a perfect pumpkin you'd serve with a roast.

Heat a glug of olive oil in a large saucepan. Add the cumin seeds, garam masala, and thyme. Stir well. You may go a little giddy with the amazing aroma crawling into your nostrils. No, it's not a bad trip, go with it.

After 5 minutes add the garlic and onion, and cook until softened (8 minutes).

Remove the pumpkin from the oven and add to the saucepan, mix well, feel free to mash it a little with a mashy thing.

Add the curry powder.

While the soup is simmering, panfry the pine nuts in olive oil until golden brown and pop the ciabatta bread in the toaster.

Now give the soup a good whiz with a stick blender until super smooth.

Simmer on low heat for 10 minutes. Season to taste.

Turn off the heat and stir in the cream.

Spread the Gorgonzola on to the toasted ciabatta and place on top of each serve of soup with a garnish of the pine nuts.

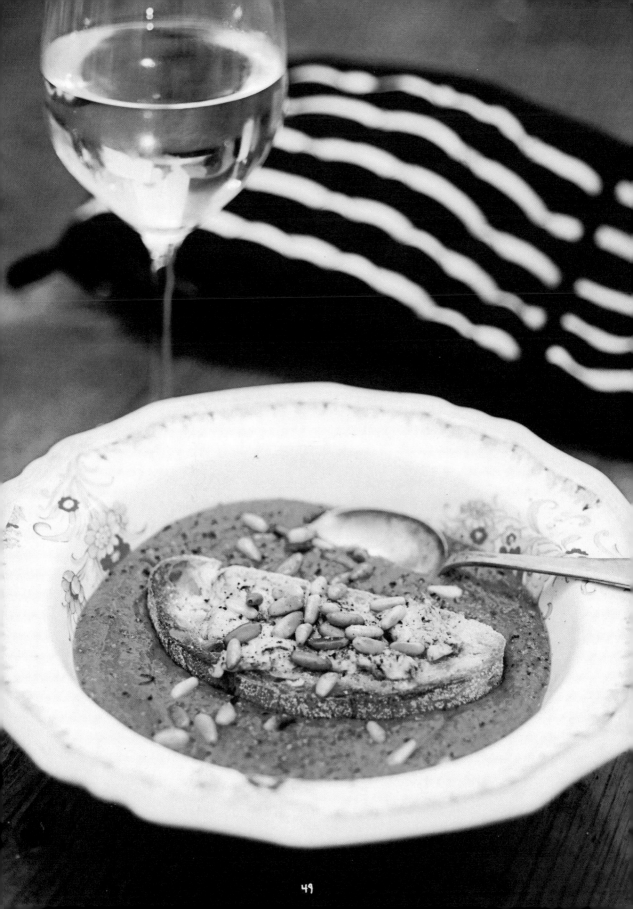

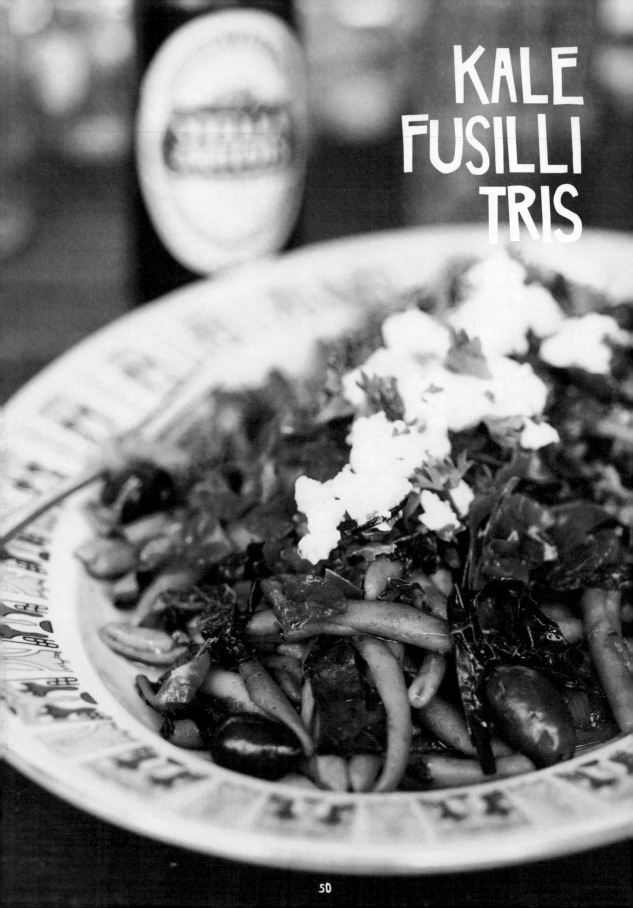

KALE
FUSILLI
TRIS

SINCE EMBRACING SEASONAL EATING, I'VE FALLEN MADLY IN LOVE WITH A FEW MEALS THAT TAKE CENTER STAGE ON MY TABLE AT CERTAIN TIMES OF THE YEAR. THEY EXIST AS A CELEBRATION OF WHAT IT IS POSSIBLE TO GROW AT THAT PARTICULAR TIME OF THE SEASON. I WON'T ARGUE THAT GROWING VEGETABLES IN WINTER IS A CHALLENGE; WITH SINGLE DIGIT TEMPERATURES, FROSTS, AND PLENTY OF MOISTURE THE PLANTS JUST DON'T FEEL MUCH LIKE GROWING! HOWEVER, THERE ARE A FEW HARDY VARIETIES THAT I'VE COME TO LOVE OVER THE COLD WINTER MONTHS.

KALE SITS HIGH ON THAT LIST. IT'S A WINTER GREEN THAT IS NOT ONLY FULL OF FLAVOR BUT IS ALSO FAIRLY DYNAMIC IN THE KITCHEN. IT CAN BE FRIED, STEAMED, AND STEWED. A FRIEND INTRODUCED ME TO IT A FEW YEARS AGO ON A COLD WINTER'S DAY AT MARKET, EXPLAINING TO ME THAT IT IS AN ITALIAN FAVORITE THAT WOULD HAPPILY GROW THROUGH THE COOLER MONTHS. INTRIGUED, AND ALWAYS ON THE LOOKOUT FOR A WINTER CROP, I SOON HAD A FEW PLANTS GROWING AS A TEST. I'VE BEEN GROWING THEM AND SINGING THEIR PRAISES EVER SINCE. THERE ARE A FEW VARIETIES OF KALE, NOTABLY BLUE KALE, TUSCAN, AND THE RUSSIAN VARIETY. GROW A FEW TYPES AND SEE WHICH WORKS FOR YOU.

WHAT YOU NEED:

6 slices pancetta, roughly chopped
1 lb (500 g) fusilli tris
1 large bunch of Tuscan kale,
    cut into strips
1 large bunch of blue kale, cut into strips
1 x onion, chopped
4 x cloves garlic, copped
1 handful of parsley, chopped
1 handful of black olives (optional)
5.25 oz (150 g) marinated goat's feta
2 cups (500 ml) passata (see page 212)
1 cup red wine
Olive oil
Salt
Pepper

HOW TO:

Heat a large pot of water (with a pinch of salt) and start the pasta cooking when the water is boiling. Fusilli can take up to 25 minutes to cook, so best to get the pasta cooking before you start cooking up the sauce.

Heat a glug of oil in a frying pan, and fry up the pancetta until crispy, when done set aside to cool.

Now, panfry the onion and garlic for at least 5 minutes, just until softened, then add the chopped kale. Cook the kale down until it is reduced to half its size while continuously stirring (approx 5 minutes).

Add the red wine, passata, olives, and parsley (leaving a small amount for garnish). Turn the heat down to a gentle simmer, and simmer for a further 15 minutes reducing the sauce.

Taste the sauce and season if needed. The pancetta, feta, and olives are all very salty so don't overdo the seasoning. I don't usually season this dish at all.

When the pasta is cooked al dente, drain and return it to the pot it was cooked in.

Pour in the sauce and stir well.

Serve with a generous crumble of the crispy fried pancetta, and a crumble of the feta as well.

Garnish with chopped parsley, and dress with good quality olive oil.

MINUS A FEW INGREDIENTS, THIS MEAL COMES COMPLETELY
FROM URBAN BACKYARD PRODUCE: OUR VEGETABLES,
HERBS, HOMEMADE OLIVE OIL, AND HOME-CURED CHORIZO.
I'LL NORMALLY HAVE THIS ON TOASTED BREAD FOR A
BREAKFAST MEAL, BUT IT CAN BE CONSUMED ANY
TIME OF THE DAY, AND TASTES JUST AS GOOD, IF NOT
BETTER, A DAY LATER AS LEFTOVERS.

IF YOU USE BEANS THAT YOU'VE GROWN OVER THE
SUMMER AND DRIED OUT FOR WINTER USE, THEN
REMEMBER TO SOAK THEM IN WATER OVERNIGHT AND
THEN SET ASIDE HALF AN HOUR (TO AN HOUR,
DEPENDING ON DESIRED SOFTNESS) TO BOIL THEM
BEFORE YOU START COOKING THE MEAL. IF YOU
DON'T GROW THE BEANS, USE THE TINNED OPTION,
WHICH CAN BE USED IMMEDIATELY AND DON'T
REQUIRE SOAKING.

IF YOU'RE NOT A FAN OF KALE, THEN YOU
CAN SUBSTITUTE WITH SPINACH.

GARDENER'S REWARD BREAKFAST

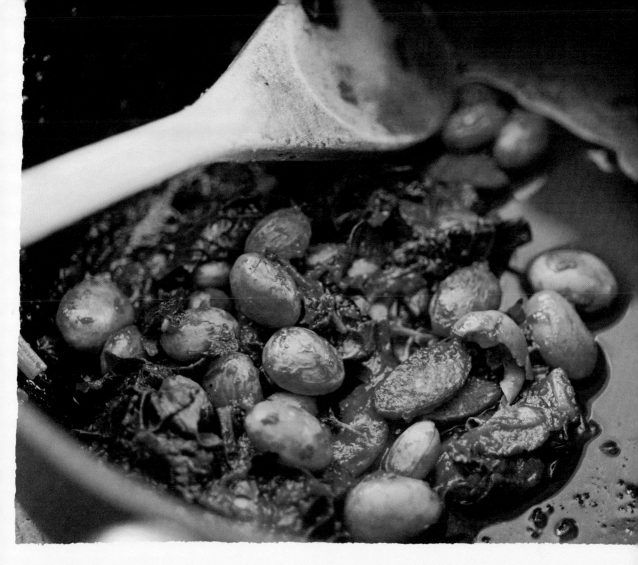

WHAT YOU NEED:

1 x chorizo sausage, chopped
3.5 oz (100 g) dried cannellini beans,
    soaked overnight and boiled until soft
Handful mixed kale, chopped
Handful baby spinach, chopped
5 x cloves garlic, diced
1 x chili, chopped, seeds removed
3 cups passata (see page 212)
Bunch of parsley, chopped
1 tbsp smoked paprika
Olive oil
Salt
Pepper

HOW TO:

Heat a glug of olive oil in a frying pan (medium to high heat). When hot, add the chorizo and brown for a few minutes, which will release the animal fats (aka "flavor").

Now add the kale and spinach, stir and toss for over 5 minutes or until the greens have reduced in size.

Add the beans, chili, paprika, passata, garlic, and chopped parsley and reduce to simmer for 10 minutes. Season with salt and pepper.

Serve on crusty toasted bread, dress with olive oil, garnish with parsley, and season.

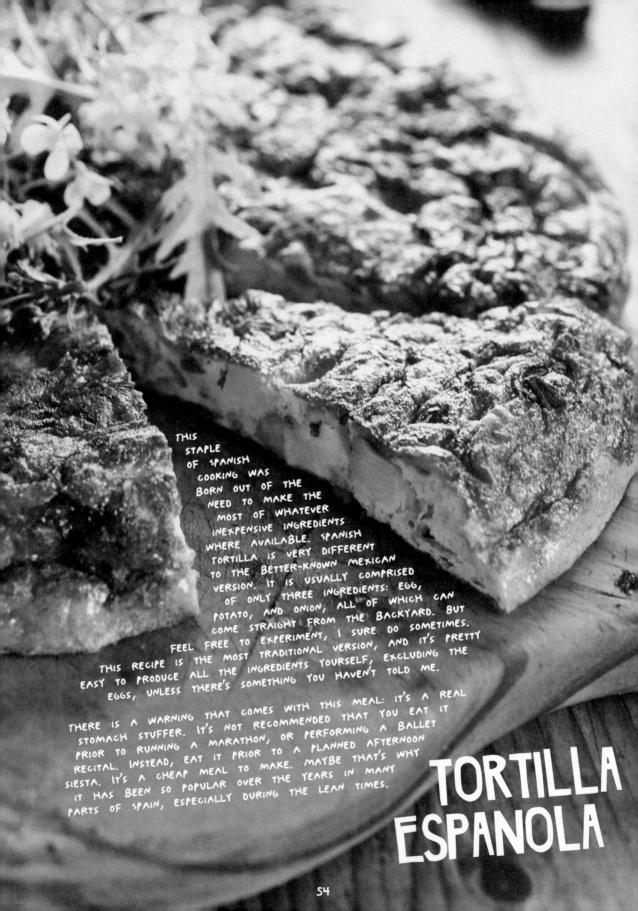

THIS
STAPLE
OF SPANISH
COOKING WAS
BORN OUT OF THE
NEED TO MAKE THE
MOST OF WHATEVER
INEXPENSIVE INGREDIENTS
WHERE AVAILABLE. SPANISH
TORTILLA IS VERY DIFFERENT
TO THE BETTER-KNOWN MEXICAN
VERSION. IT IS USUALLY COMPRISED
OF ONLY THREE INGREDIENTS: EGG,
POTATO, AND ONION, ALL OF WHICH CAN
COME STRAIGHT FROM THE BACKYARD. BUT
FEEL FREE TO EXPERIMENT, I SURE DO SOMETIMES.
THIS RECIPE IS THE MOST TRADITIONAL VERSION, AND IT'S PRETTY
EASY TO PRODUCE ALL THE INGREDIENTS YOURSELF, EXCLUDING THE
EGGS, UNLESS THERE'S SOMETHING YOU HAVEN'T TOLD ME.

THERE IS A WARNING THAT COMES WITH THIS MEAL: IT'S A REAL
STOMACH STUFFER. IT'S NOT RECOMMENDED THAT YOU EAT IT
PRIOR TO RUNNING A MARATHON, OR PERFORMING A BALLET
RECITAL. INSTEAD, EAT IT PRIOR TO A PLANNED AFTERNOON
SIESTA. IT'S A CHEAP MEAL TO MAKE. MAYBE THAT'S WHY
IT HAS BEEN SO POPULAR OVER THE YEARS IN MANY
PARTS OF SPAIN, ESPECIALLY DURING THE LEAN TIMES.

TORTILLA ESPANOLA

WHAT YOU NEED:

6-7 x eggs
6 x medium potatoes
2 x onions, sliced
Olive oil

HOW TO:

Preheat the oven to 400 F (200 C).

Peel the potatoes and parboil for 10 minutes. Allow them to cool and then slice in half lengthwise, then with the flat side down, slice them into small chunks about 3/4 in (2 cm) long.

In a frying pan, heat a good glug of olive oil (at least 1/4 cup). To test if the oil is at the correct cooking temperature, place in one slice of potato, when it sizzles it's ready to go.

Cook the potato and onion for about five minutes, until the color starts to turn.

Remove the onion and potato from the pan and drain off any excess oil using a colander, and allow to cool.

In a large mixing bowl, combine the eggs, paprika, and the fried onion and potato. Mix well.

Heat a large frying pan to medium heat, but not hot, so you won't burn the eggs.

Mix all the ingredients one last time before pouring onto the medium heat frying pan. Do not mix in the pan; just allow it to cook as one piece.

Allow the mixture to cook until you can peel away the side of the tortilla from the pan with a knife. Do this to check if the sides are cooked and holding together well after about 5 minutes.

Place the pan in the oven for 15-20 minutes.

When you're ready to serve, place a cutting board or large plate over the pan. Then flip the pan over and the tortilla will slide out, in one piece, totally cooked.

Serve with a light garden salad.

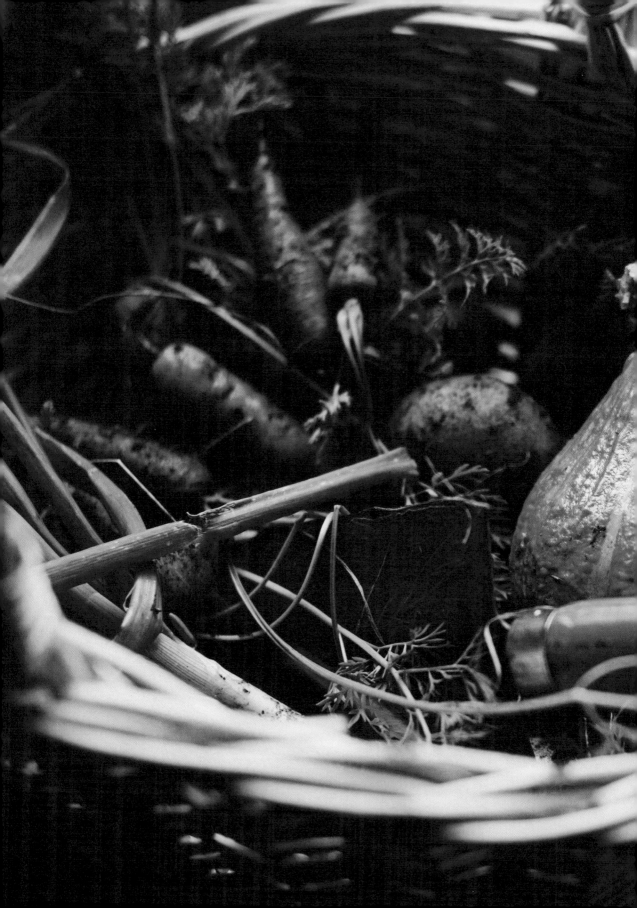

IT'S THE CYCLES OF THE GARDEN THAT KEEP ME INSPIRED.

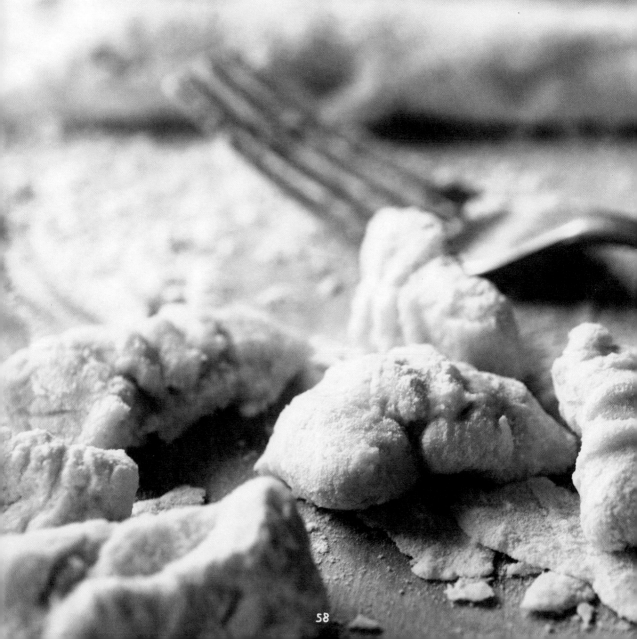

TWO-CHEESE GNOCCHI

THIS IS PRETTY RICH AND A TAD EVIL. IF YOU'RE ON A WEIGHT LOSS DIET, IMMEDIATELY TURN TO ANOTHER PAGE...ACTUALLY, PUT THE BOOK DOWN AND WALK AWAY BACKWARDS AVOIDING DIRECT EYE CONTACT. BUT IF YOU WANT YOUR MOUTH TO HAVE SOME SORT OF ORGASMIC EXPERIENCE, CONTINUE READING.

GNOCCHI IS PRETTY EASY TO MAKE AND IT'S A GREAT WAY TO COOK THE POTATOES YOU'VE GROWN. IT DOES INVOLVE A HEAP OF MESSY FLOUR AND ROLLING THINGS INTO SAUSAGE LIKE SHAPES, SO KIDS ARE DRAWN TO THE PROCESS LIKE HIPSTERS TO A SALE ON BOAT SHOES. ONCE YOU'VE MADE YOUR OWN GNOCCHI IT BECOMES VERY HARD TO BUY IT PRE-MADE—IT JUST ISN'T AS GOOD. MAKING YOUR OWN GIVES YOU A SENSE OF ACHIEVEMENT IN THE KITCHEN; A REWARD THAT YOU NEED WHEN THE REST OF YOUR DAY SEEMS TO HAVE FALLEN APART. MAKE IT! DON'T BE SCARED, I'LL HOLD YOUR HAND. OH, IT'S COVERED IN FLOUR AND MASHED POTATOES? HOW 'BOUT WE JUST SMILE IN ACKNOWLEDGEMENT AT ONE ANOTHER.

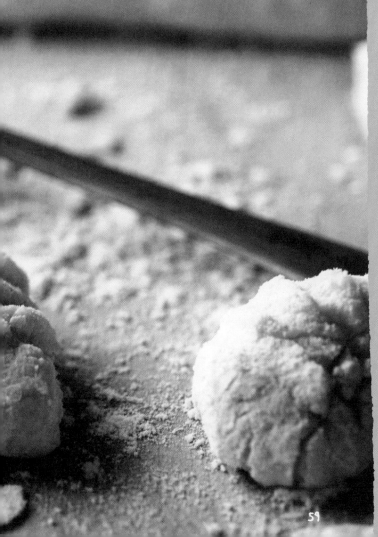

WHAT YOU NEED:

The Gnocchi
6 x potatoes, washed
1 x egg
1 x nutmeg or grated nutmeg
Plain flour
Pepper, grated

The Evil Sauce
1 cup pecorino cheese, grated
5.25 oz (150 g) Gorgonzola cheese
Knob of butter

HOW TO:

Make basic gnocchi (see page 231). Boil them.

Place a large frying pan on low/medium heat. Add a knob of butter and the Gorgonzola.

After a few minutes the gnocchi will start to float to the surface of the boiling water indicating they're cooked. Scoop out with a straining spoon and add to the frying pan, mixing very gently as the fresh gnocchi is very fragile. It's best (if you can) to give the pan constant "chef flicks" to coat the gnocchi well, instead of using a mixing spoon. Add the pecorino cheese, season, and stir well.

If you're convinced it's not as indulgent as it should be, add some shredded, crispy-cooked prosciutto as a garnish.

PUMPKIN GNOCCHI

THE ONLY THING THIS GNOCCHI SHARES WITH A POTATO GNOCCHI IS TEXTURE— THE FLAVORS ARE TOTALLY DIFFERENT. IN WINTER, WHEN NOT MUCH IS KEEPING THE GARDEN GREEN, THE STORED PUMPKIN BECOMES A RELIABLE SOURCE OF VEG. AT THE END OF SUMMER WHEN THE PUMPKIN PLANT STARTS TO DIE BACK, LEAVE THE PUMPKIN ON THE VINE UNTIL THE PLANT IS TOTALLY DEAD, AND THEN CUT IT OFF LEAVING AT LEAST 6 INCHES (15 CM) OF THE STEM STILL ATTACHED. THIS HELPS INCREASE THE PUMPKIN'S STORAGE VIABILITY THROUGH WINTER. EVEN THOUGH THIS MEAL IS FAIRLY BASIC, IT HAS REAL POTENTIAL TO IMPRESS THE HECK OUT OF YOUR GUESTS.

WHAT YOU NEED:

Gnocchi:

- 1 x pumpkin, skinned and deseeded (potimarron or butternut sized)
- 1 x egg
- 1 x nutmeg, grated
- Plain flour
- Semolina
- Cracked black pepper
- Olive oil

Sauce:

- 4 strips prosciutto, chopped
- 1 bunch fresh basil, chopped
- 3.5 oz (100 g) marinated goat's feta
- 1/4 cup (50 g) pouring cream
- 3/4 cup (100 g) pine nuts
- Parmesan
- Olive oil
- Salt
- Pepper

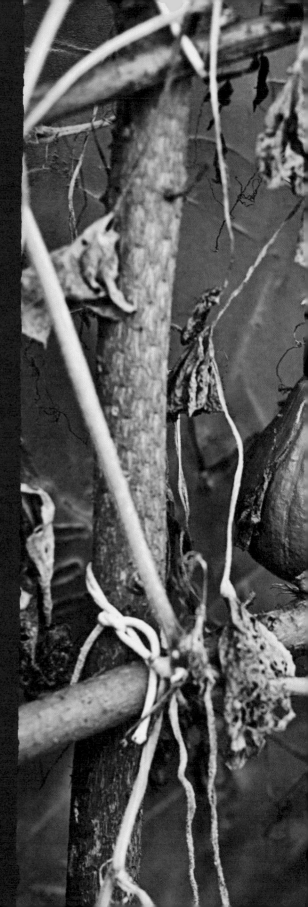

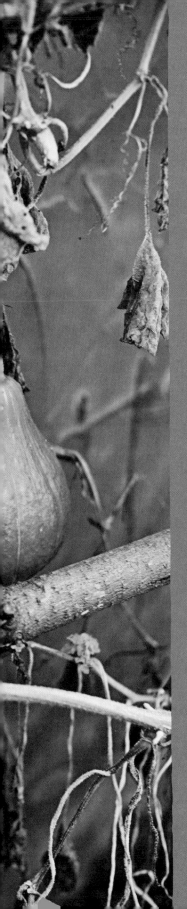

HOW TO:

Preheat the oven to 400 F (200 C).

Cut the pumpkin into large chunks and place in a large baking dish. Generously drizzle with oil and toss well to ensure each piece has a light dressing of oil.

Bake for half an hour, or until you can easily pierce the pumpkin with a skewer.

Remove pumpkin from the oven and allow to rest until its cool enough to handle.

Place the pumpkin in a large mixing bowl, crack in some black pepper, and grate half a nutmeg into the mix. Then add the egg and stir well with a large wooden spoon.

Cover your kitchen bench with flour, and dust your hands with flour.

Pour out the mix onto the bench and start kneading until you have a strong dough that holds together well. Add more flour as needed.

Separate the dough into smaller sections and roll them out into long sausage shapes about 1 in (2-3 cm) thick.

Cut small gnocchi, about 1 in (2-3cm) long. Two options to pretty-up the gnocchi, at this point are to either roll each gnocchi over the end of a fork, leaving an indentation, or press the gnocchi down on a flat surface while rolling your thumb at the same time, to make a thumbprint indentation. There are no hard and fast rules, so feel free to play around with different methods of your own devising.

Once you have all your gnocchi made, place it on trays that have been dusted with semolina. Place in the fridge for a few hours to help them to hold their shape when they cook.

When you're ready to make the dish, heat a frying pan on medium heat and brown the pine nuts and prosciutto in glug of olive oil. When browned, set aside to cool.

Boil some salted water and cook the gnocchi. Because it's fresh it won't take long to cook. You can tell when they're cooked when the gnocchi float to the surface.

Scoop out the gnocchi into a large mixing bowl as it rises to the surface.

Add the pine nuts, prosciutto, pouring cream, and fresh basil. Stir well.

Serve with a garnish of the marinated feta, shaved Parmesan, fresh basil, and dress with olive oil.

ROAST CAPSICUM DIP

WHAT YOU NEED:

4 x red capsicums
1 x clove garlic
3.5 oz (100 g) Philadelphia
   cream cheese
3.5 oz (100 g) feta cheese
1 handful fresh basil, chopped
Salt
Pepper

HOW TO:

Preheat your oven to 400 F
(200 C).

Deseed and roughly chop the
capsicum into quarters.

Place the capsicum in an oven
dish and coat and toss with
olive oil. Roast for 35 minutes.

Allow the capsicum to cool and
whiz it in a food processor.

Add the cheese, basil, and garlic
and whiz well. Season to taste.

Pour mix into ramekins and put
in the fridge at least 2 hours
prior to serving.

Spread over toasted ciabatta or
crackers.

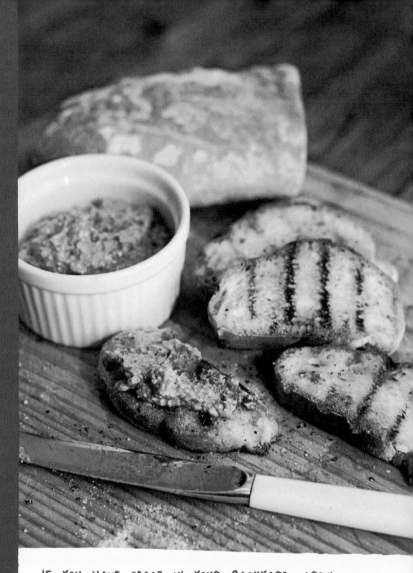

IF YOU HAVE SPACE IN YOUR BACKYARD, GROW CAPSICUMS! EVEN IF YOU HAVE A DECENT SIZE POT ON YOUR APARTMENT VERANDA YOU CAN GROW A CAPSICUM PLANT OVER THE SUMMER MONTHS. LIKE TOMATOES THEY EMBODY THE TASTE OF SUMMER, AND PERSONALLY I THINK THEY HAVE A BEAUTY ALL THEIR OWN. SURE, YOU CAN USE THEM IN SALADS, STEWS, AND ON THE BBQ. BUT THIS DIP IS A LITTLE BIT FANCIER WAY OF EATING THEM—WITH THE ADDED BONUS OF GETTING TO PRETEND THAT YOU'RE GETTING YOUR SERVINGS OF VEGETABLES FOR THE DAY (JUST IGNORE THE AMOUNT OF CHEESE YOU USED TO MAKE IT).

ROASTING THE CAPSICUMS BRINGS OUT THAT SMOKINESS THAT TRULY MAKES THE DIP. I PREFER TO USE SUPER RIPE RED CAPSICUMS, BUT YOU CAN USE GREEN, PURPLE AND YELLOW AND THE DOMINANT COLOR WILL REMAIN IN THE DIP. BE ADVENTUROUS THOUGH, PLAY AROUND AND GROW DIFFERENT TYPES. LIKE ALL VEGGIES THERE SEEMS TO BE A LIMITLESS VARIETY OF SEEDS TO BUY ONLINE.

PUMPKIN DIP

WHAT YOU NEED:

1 x pumpkin (potimarron or butternut)
3/4 cup (100 g) pine nuts
5.25 oz (150 g) feta cheese
Pecorino cheese
1 handful fresh basil
Olive oil
Salt
Pepper

HOW TO:

Preheat the oven to 350 F (180 C).

Slice the pumpkin into chunks, cut off the skin, and place in a large oven-baking dish. Coat and toss with olive oil.

Bake for 30 minutes, or until the pumpkin can be pierced easily using a fork. When the pumpkin is cooked, set it aside to cool.

Finely chop the fresh basil and set aside.

Using a frying pan, toast the pine nuts for a few minutes in a dash of olive oil. You only need a few minutes. Try not to burn them. Stir often.

Transfer the pine nuts into a food processor and whiz well, then add the pumpkin, more whizzing, then crumble in the feta and finally add the basil.

Season with salt and pepper.

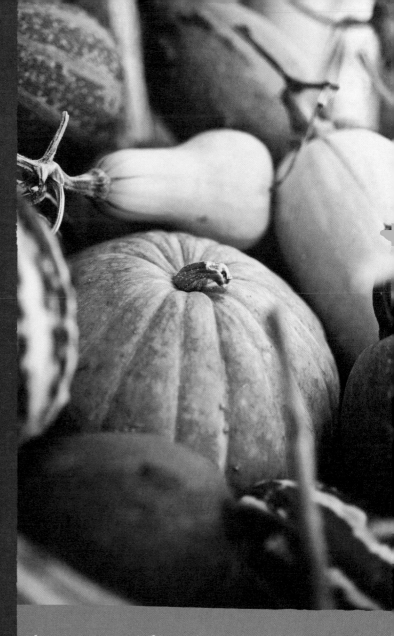

ROASTING PUMPKIN BRINGS OUT ITS SWEETNESS ALONG WITH THAT CHAR-GRILLED FLAVOR THAT WORKS REALLY WELL WITH TOASTED PINE NUTS. ONCE I STARTED TO MAKE MY OWN DIPS, I COULD NEVER UNDERSTAND WHY PEOPLE BUY THE PREMADE ONES AT SUPERMARKETS. YOU CAN HAVE SO MUCH FUN MAKING YOUR OWN, AND ITS EVEN MORE REWARDING USING YOUR OWN PRODUCE. ALL IT TAKES IS A FEW EXTRA INGREDIENTS TO COMPLEMENT YOUR VEGGIES AND VOILA! A DIP THAT IS SURE TO IMPRESS ANYONE. THE FLAVORS ARE SURE TO SURPASS THE SHELVED VARIETIES. WHEN USING VEGETABLES THAT YOU'VE GROWN YOURSELF, IT ALWAYS TASTES BETTER.

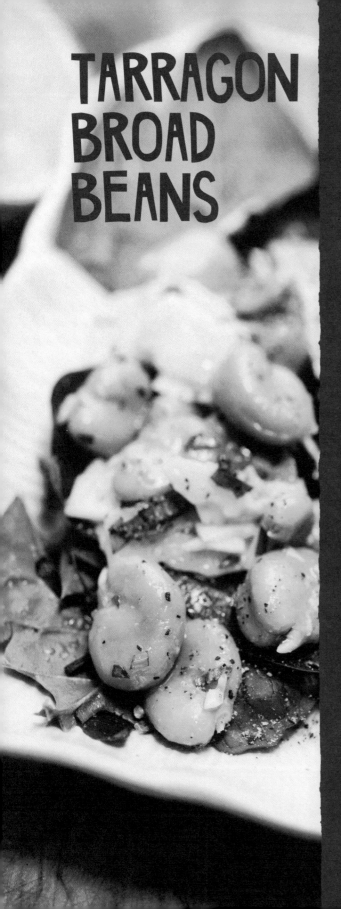

TARRAGON BROAD BEANS

EACH WINTER IT'S ADVISABLE TO PLANT A GREEN MULCH CROP LIKE MUSTARD OR BROAD BEANS, WHICH, AS A BI-PRODUCT OF THEIR GROWTH, REPLENISH THE NITROGEN LEVELS OF THE SOIL. FOR YEARS I'D BEEN GROWING THE BEANS AND THEN DIGGING THEM INTO THE SOIL AS GREEN MULCH ABOUT A MONTH PRIOR TO PLANTING TOMATOES. BUT THEN AFTER SOME ENCOURAGEMENT FROM A POLISH FRIEND, I STARTED EATING THEM IN VARIOUS RECIPES. LO AND BEHOLD, I NO LONGER VIEWED THEM AS JUST ANOTHER GREEN MULCH.

THIS IS A SUMMER TREAT, A SIMPLE TAPA, SOMETHING TO BE SHARED ON THE TABLE OR USED AS A SIDE BEAN SALAD.

WHAT YOU NEED:

1 large handful fresh broad beans
1 x lemon
1 small bunch fresh tarragon
Parmesan cheese
Olive Oil
Salt
Pepper

HOW TO:

Remove the beans from the pods, and blanch in a pot of boiling water for 5 minutes.

Drain and allow to cool.

While the beans are cooling, shave some good quality Parmesan cheese.

Finely chop the tarragon. Set aside.

Place the beans in a mixing bowl, grate over the rind of the lemon, and then squeeze the lemon juice in.

Add the tarragon, dress with olive oil, season with salt and pepper, and when plating up, garnish with a healthy serving of the Parmesan cheese.

CHAR-GRILLED EGGPLANT DIP

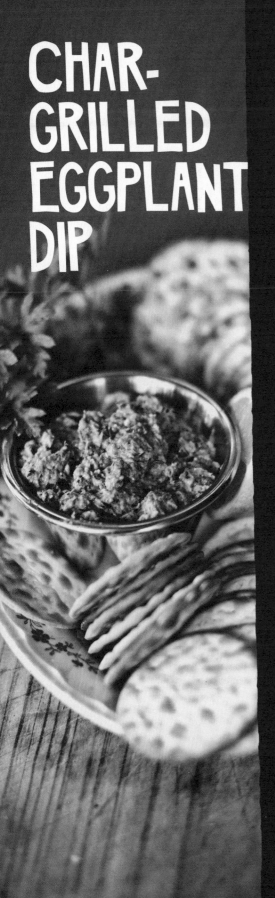

EGGPLANT IS ONE OF MY FAVORITE SUMMER VEGETABLES TO GROW. IT'S A LOT LIKE ZUCCHINI IN THAT ONCE THE WARM WEATHER ARRIVES IT REALLY GETS A WRIGGLE ON. THERE IS A GREAT RANGE OF EGGPLANT VARIETIES FROM SHORT STUMPY ONES TO LONG AND SLENDER AND EVEN ZEBRA STRIPPED (WHICH STARTS TO SOUND LIKE A RANGE OF ADULT TOYS).

CHAR-GRILLING EGGPLANT BRINGS OUT THAT GREAT SMOKY ROASTED FLAVOR, AND GRILLED EGGPLANT ON ITS OWN IS PERFECT WITH SOME FETA, MARINATED CAPSICUM, AND FRIED MUSHROOM ALL TOASTED BETWEEN A COUPLE SLICES OF FOCACCIA. BUT THIS RECIPE TAKES IT ONE STEP FURTHER, MAKING IT INTO A DIP THAT IS A REAL TREAT ON TOASTED CIABATTA OR WITH WATER CRACKERS.

WHAT YOU NEED:

2 x eggplant
1 x fresh chili (de-seeded)
5 x cloves garlic
3.5 oz (100 g) feta cheese
1 tbsp red wine vinegar
1 tbsp tahini
1 bunch fresh parsley
1/2 tsp cumin
Olive oil
Salt
Pepper

HOW TO:

Slice the eggplant lengthways (skin on) and place on a tray.

Finely chop the fresh parsley, chili, and the garlic.

Sprinkle each layer of sliced eggplant with some salt and a generous drizzle of olive oil.

Use either a BBQ grill or a griddle pan to grill the eggplant until soft.

Place all the grilled eggplant into a food processer and whiz well.

Add the feta, tahini, chopped parsley, garlic, red wine vinegar, and chili, and season with salt and pepper.

Transfer into a bowl and refrigerate for and few hours before serving.

GEAR

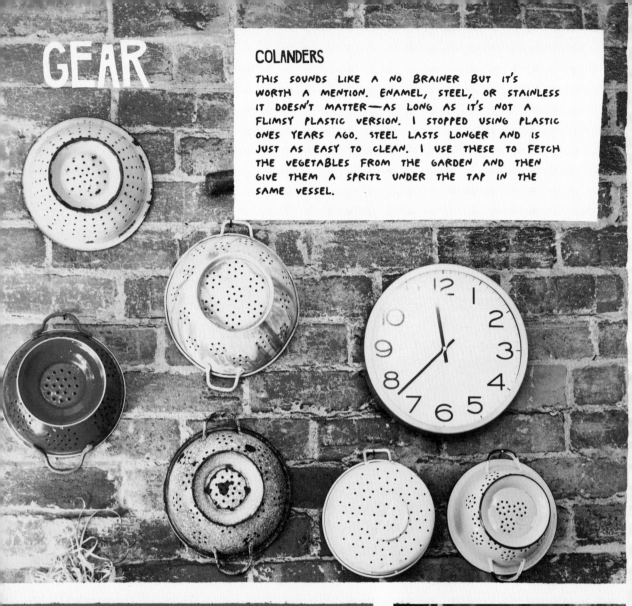

COLANDERS

THIS SOUNDS LIKE A NO BRAINER BUT IT'S WORTH A MENTION. ENAMEL, STEEL, OR STAINLESS IT DOESN'T MATTER—AS LONG AS IT'S NOT A FLIMSY PLASTIC VERSION. I STOPPED USING PLASTIC ONES YEARS AGO. STEEL LASTS LONGER AND IS JUST AS EASY TO CLEAN. I USE THESE TO FETCH THE VEGETABLES FROM THE GARDEN AND THEN GIVE THEM A SPRITZ UNDER THE TAP IN THE SAME VESSEL.

TROWEL

ONCE A GARDEN HAS BEEN DUG OVER ONCE AND YOU KEEP THE SOIL NICE AND FRIABLE WITH PLENTY OF ORGANIC MATTER AND MULCH, THE ONLY SHOVEL YOU REALLY NEED IS A SMALL TROWEL. IT DOES EVERYTHING I NEED IT TO. IT'S USEFUL WHEN WEEDING, WHEN DIGGING OVER NEW MANURE, AND MAKING ROWS AND HOLES TO PLANT NEW CROPS. INSTEAD OF HAVING A SHED FULL OF TOOLS I LIKE TO USE A SELECT FEW, AND A WOOD-HANDLED, STEEL-NOSE TROWEL IS A GO. AS WITH ANY GARDEN TOOL WITH A WOODEN HANDLE, OCCASIONALLY USE LIGHT SAND PAPER TO REMOVE SPLINTERS AND RUB IT DOWN WITH LINSEED OIL TO MAINTAIN LONGEVITY. LOOK AFTER YOUR TOOLS AND THEY'LL LOOK AFTER YOU.

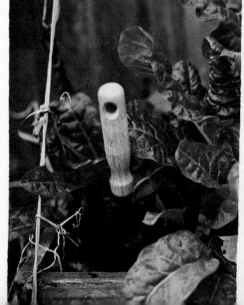

LEATHER SLIP-ON BOOTS

A GENERAL-PURPOSE GARDENING AND WORKMAN'S BOOT. STEEL-CAPPED TOES ARE A GOOD OPTION IF YOU'RE CLUMSY. AUSTRALIAN-MADE BLUNDSTONE BOOTS ARE UNBEATABLE FOR THIS PURPOSE, DESIGNED AND MADE WITH ONE INTENTION: TO SURVIVE RUGGED TREATMENT FROM AUSSIE "TRADIES" (TRADESMEN, BUILDERS, PLUMBERS, ETC.).

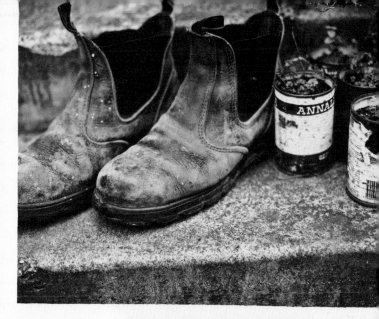

VEST

I PICKED UP A WORKMAN'S VEST THAT'S LINED WITH DUCK DOWN, AND I LOVE IT. IT'S MY MOST WORN GARMENT. IT LEAVES MY ARMS FREE FOR GARDENING, FISHING, AND HUNTING, WHERE A JACKET WOULD BE RESTRICTIVE. CARHARTT IS THE BOMB.

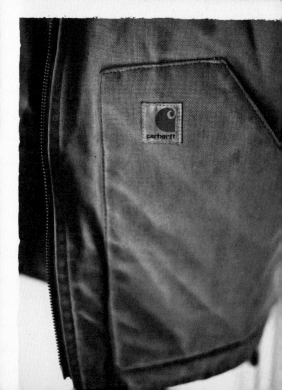

WATERING CAN

I KNOW WHAT YEAR IT IS. I KNOW I COULD SET UP AN AUTOMATED WATERING SYSTEM. BUT THE FACT IS I JUST DON'T WANT TO. I ENJOY USING A METAL WATERING CAN; IT FORCES ME TO SLOW DOWN AND TAKE THE TIME TO ADMIRE THE PLANTS. YES I'M A HIPPIE. I LIKE A CAN THAT'S STURDY AND BUILT TO LAST A LONG TIME. PLASTIC FEELS CHEAP, METAL IS BEST.

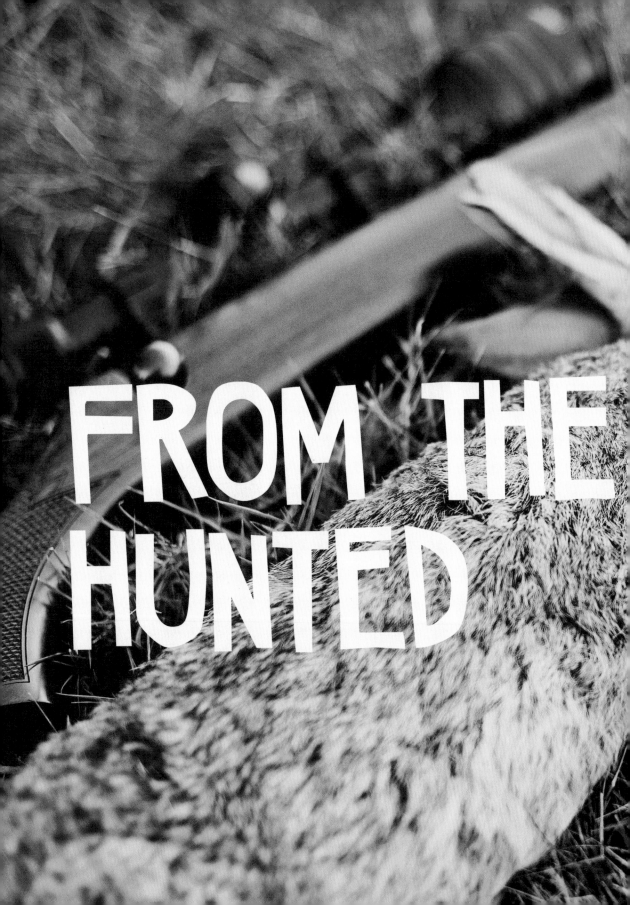

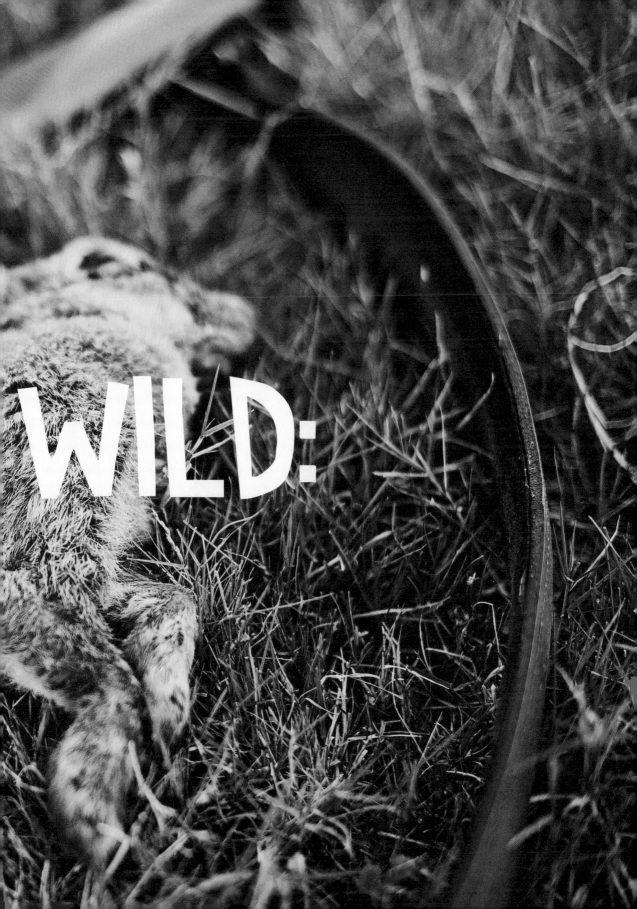

WILD:

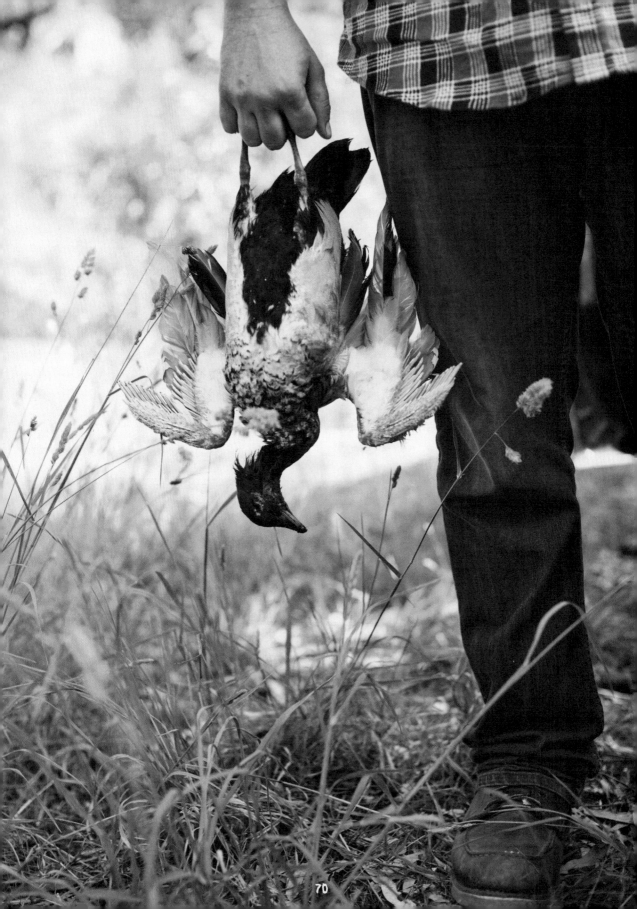

Some countries accept hunting as a legitimate approach to sourcing meat. Others do not. It's a complex issue that I don't want to go into too much—I might end up pulling my hair out in frustration, so I'll leave politics aside. Suffice to say that, in my view, hunting within your region in sustainable quantities is completely acceptable. Hunting for food is clearly different than hunting for sport, the latter of which I don't really understand (to each their own I suppose).

Nature is very clever. It has ways of controlling population numbers without our intervention. I know, amazing right?! When weather conditions are good and food is plentiful, there's a heavy breeding season; alternatively when food is scarce, so too is population growth. It makes sense to take meat from the wild. It's healthy, fresh, and the animals have lived a free and natural existence— unlike the dark and dirty poultry farms that supply the Western world's hunger for cheap chicken, or the frightful, massive, large-scale cattle and hog farms. Brrrr!

Some might argue that if everyone started hunting then we'd demolish the natural populations of game to oblivion. This is clearly never going to happen as most of the Western world lives in major cities and there just isn't the inclination to hunt. Most people would understand that to hunt requires a fair bit of practice and know-how; it's not just a matter of grabbing a gun and sharpshooting like Wyatt Earp.

If you want to start hunting with a rifle, or even a bow for that matter, the first step is to check your local and state laws. Most governing bodies will have a website that can inform you of the steps you will need to take to obtain a hunting license (and how to legally acquire and carry a firearm). In my state you attend a mandatory safety course, take a test, then, if you're approved, you can apply for a firearm permit.

Suddenly you find yourself a gun owner who can legally fire a weapon, but you might never have fired a gun in your life. Luckily for me, I had some shooting experience growing up on a farm, but for many people it's a new experience. If you know someone who does use firearms for hunting, ask them if they'd mind taking you out to show you the basics. I once took a friend out for a shoot with a .22 magnum and let him hunt his first small game. He later admitted that he was initially anxious about the whole process but after it was all done he had a completely different view and respect for how meat is obtained. I later handed him a 12-gauge shotgun and watched him almost get bowled over from the recoil. He didn't enjoy that part of the experience so much.

If you don't know an experienced shooter who you can learn from, don't panic, there are alternatives. You can join a gun club or go to a shooting range for some experience. At these places there will be plenty of knowledgeable shooters to share their experience and expertise, and no doubt a few wankers, too (avoid them at all costs). Remember, guns are designed to inflict mortal injury. Safety is key both in regard to usage and storage. However, if they are handled appropriately, they're extremely useful tools.

Some people use dogs, some people shoot out of the back of a pickup, and some people sit and stalk. All methods have varying levels of success and all are determined to some extent by to the type of game you're hunting. Again, utilize hunting or shooting clubs to learn the ropes.

Hunting is my way of viscerally connecting with the need to source my own meat. I can't deny that it is something primeval. It's satisfying knowing that I can source meat from the wild. I can survive off the land. That's why hunting is a skill common to people who live in rural communities. It's a connection to nature.

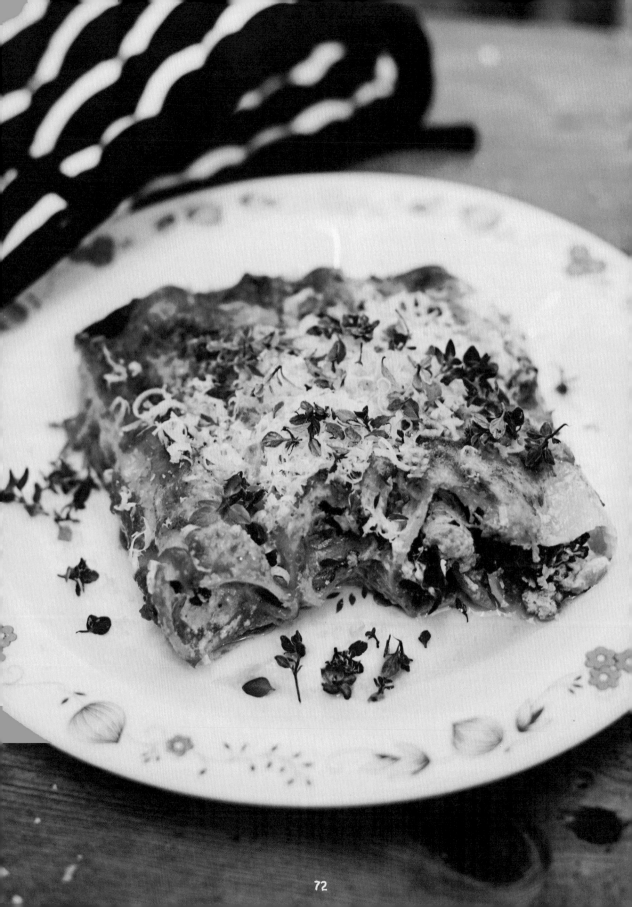

FURRED GAME + KALE CANNELLONI

THIS IS A REAL SHOWSTOPPER; A FAVORITE FOR OUR BROOD AS THE COOLER WEATHER SETS IN. IT'S A BIT OF A FIDDLE TO MAKE, BUT IF YOU GET YOUR FRIENDS TO SIT AROUND THE TABLE WITH YOU, THEY WILL GIVE YOU PLENTY OF UNWANTED ADVICE AS YOU STUFF THE CANNELLONI, WHICH HELPS TO PASS THE TIME.

POACHING FURRED GAME SUCH AS RABBIT AND HARE IS VERY EASY. JUST POP THE BUNNY IN BOILING WATER FOR TWO HOURS, MAKING SURE THAT AT ALL TIMES THE MEAT IS IN THE WATER (YOU MAY NEED TO WEIGH IT DOWN). ALLOW THE BODY TO COOL THEN REMOVE THE MEAT FROM THE BONE.

WHAT YOU NEED:

1 x whole rabbit or hare, poached for
    2 hours, meat removed (see page 103)
1/2 lb (250 g) cannelloni pasta
1 bunch of brown kale, chopped
1 bunch of black kale, chopped
6 x cloves garlic, chopped
1 x onion, chopped
14 oz (400 g) ricotta
Mozzarella
Parmesan cheese, grated
Small tub of cream
1 bunch fresh thyme
    (set some aside for garnish)
1 bunch fresh parsley
Nutmeg
Olive oil
Salt
Pepper

Sauce:
26 oz (750 ml) passata (see page 212)
1/2 cup red wine
2 tbsp red wine vinegar
1 tin chopped Italian tomatoes
Salt
Pepper

HOW TO:

Heat a frying pan and add a glug of olive oil. Panfry the garlic and onion until soft and the color has changed.

Add your chopped kale and cook until it has shrunk (around 6 minutes). Set aside in a large mixing bowl to cool.

Once cool and easy to handle, add the ricotta, poached rabbit meat (finely chopped), thyme, and parsley remembering to set aside some thyme for the garnish. Give it a good mix and set aside. This mixture will be the stuffing for your cannelloni.

To make your tomato sauce base, heat a saucepan and add all of your tomato sauce ingredients. Simmer for 10 minutes.

Preheat your oven to 400 F (200 C).

Now you can start stuffing! That mixture needs to get into those little cannelloni tubes. You can use a teaspoon, your fingers, or a baking squeeze tube. Use whatever works best for you. Fill those babies with your yummy mixture and lay them out in a baking dish. Then pour in your tomato sauce and cover them.

In a bowl, mix up your cream and a cup of grated Parmesan cheese. Once mixed well pour over the top of the pasta. Place some mozzarella on top and grate a good layer of Parmesan cheese over that to make a delicious, crusty cheese top.

Cover dish with aluminum foil and bake covered for 15 minutes at 400 F (200 C) and uncovered at 300 F (150 C) for 15 minutes.

GARDENER'S PAYBACK PAELLA

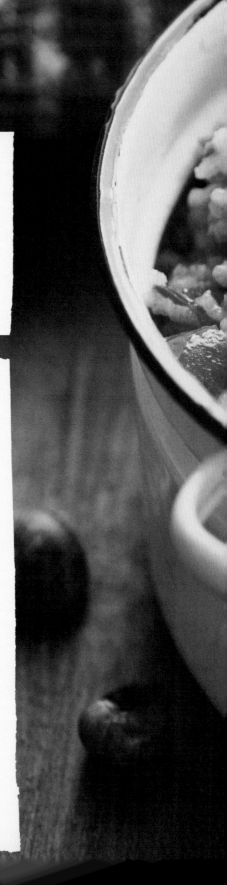

WHAT YOU NEED:

1 x whole young, wild rabbit

40-50 garden snails (selected with extreme prejudice, purged and washed)

1 x chorizo link, chopped

2 x cups Arborio rice

1 x red capsicum, de-seeded and chopped

4 x ripe tomatoes, de-seeded and chopped

5 x cloves garlic, chopped

1 cup white wine

1/2 cup Fino sherry

2 x tsp smoked paprika

2 x tsp cumin

10-15 strands saffron

Olive oil

Pepper

Salt

HOW TO:

Boil the snails for an hour in 1/2 gallon (2 liters) water.

Mash the garlic, cumin, and paprika with a mortar and pestle. Add the white wine and mix well.

Section the rabbit, first cutting off all the legs, and then chopping the body into thirds. No fixed rules here—just get the rabbit into sections so that everyone can get some meat.

When the snails have boiled for an hour, heat a large, heavy-based pot with a glug of olive oil, and cook the chopped chorizo for a few minutes to release the flavor of the sausage.

Next add the rabbit and brown it for a few minutes on each side, then pour in the Fino sherry and cook it off.

Add the snails and the liquid they were cooked in.

Add the chopped tomato, capsicum, and the saffron, and the mix from the mortar and pestle.

Make sure the meat is covered in liquid, if more is needed add warm water.

Pour in the rice and stir well to mix.

Bring to a simmer and cook for 40 minutes or until the meat falls from the bone and the rice is cooked through like a risotto.

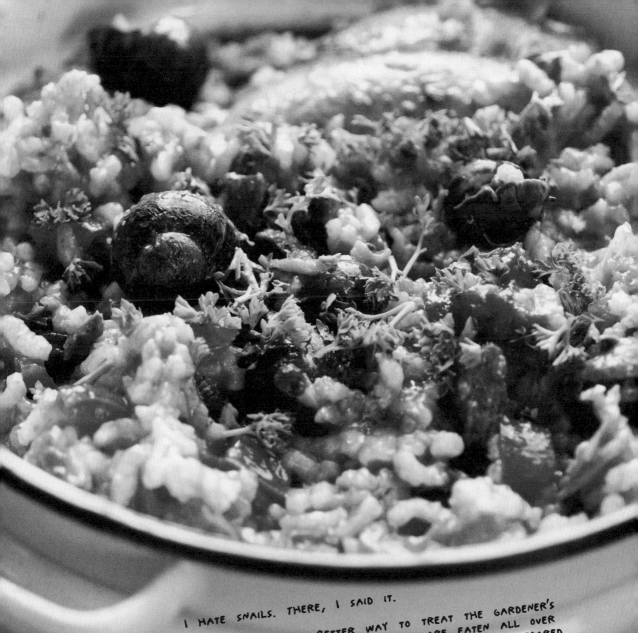

I HATE SNAILS. THERE, I SAID IT.

I COULDN'T THINK OF A BETTER WAY TO TREAT THE GARDENER'S MOST HATED PEST THAN TO EAT IT. SNAILS ARE EATEN ALL OVER THE WORLD, AND WHY NOT? THEY TASTE GOOD (ESPECIALLY PREPARED AS THE RENOWNED ESCARGOT). IT'S JUST OUR OPPRESSED AND SELECTIVE WESTERN UPBRINGING THAT PROGRAMS OUR MINDS REGARDING WHAT IS ACCEPTABLE FOOD AND WHAT IS NOT. IT'S CLEAR THAT OUR PRIVILEGE OFTEN KEEPS US FROM EATING "ALTERNATIVE" FORMS OF FOOD, BUT WEIRDER THINGS ARE EATEN IN COUNTRIES ALL OVER THE WORLD.

PICK YOUR SNAILS ON A RAINY NIGHT. WANDER IN THE YARD WITH A TORCH AND BUCKET, IMAGINE WHAT THE NEIGHBORS WILL THINK (IT'S ADVISED TO NOT APPEAR TO BE DIGGING SHALLOW GRAVES IN THE YARD). STORE THE SNAILS IN AN AERATED, SEALED PLASTIC TUB, FEED THEM WASHED LETTUCE, AND PURGE THEM FOR A WEEK TO REMOVE ANY TOXINS. WHEN YOU'RE ABOUT TO COOK THEM WASH THEM IN A BOWL OF COLD WATER.

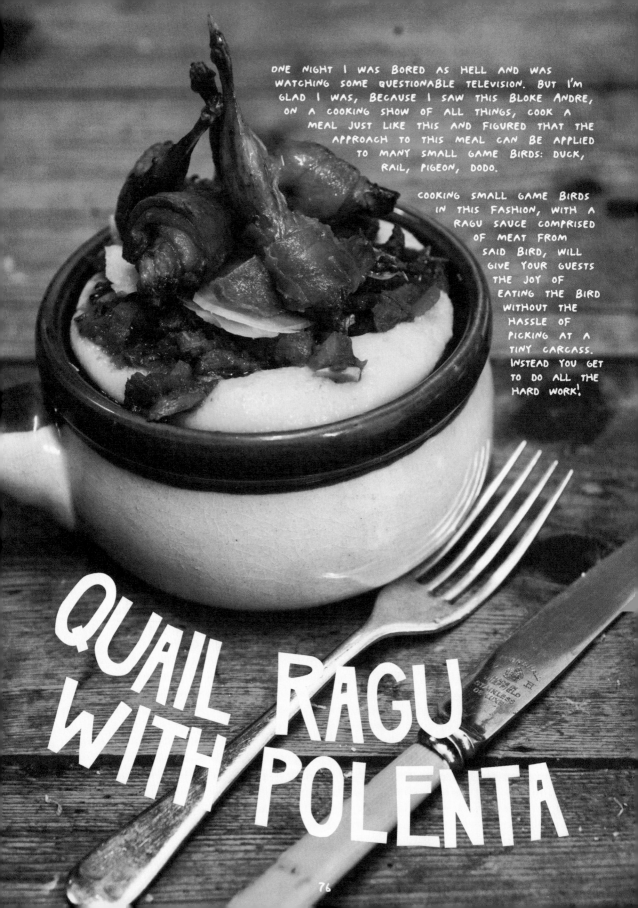

ONE NIGHT I WAS BORED AS HELL AND WAS WATCHING SOME QUESTIONABLE TELEVISION. BUT I'M GLAD I WAS, BECAUSE I SAW THIS BLOKE ANDRE, ON A COOKING SHOW OF ALL THINGS, COOK A MEAL JUST LIKE THIS AND FIGURED THAT THE APPROACH TO THIS MEAL CAN BE APPLIED TO MANY SMALL GAME BIRDS: DUCK, RAIL, PIGEON, DODO.

COOKING SMALL GAME BIRDS IN THIS FASHION, WITH A RAGU SAUCE COMPRISED OF MEAT FROM SAID BIRD, WILL GIVE YOUR GUESTS THE JOY OF EATING THE BIRD WITHOUT THE HASSLE OF PICKING AT A TINY CARCASS. INSTEAD YOU GET TO DO ALL THE HARD WORK!

QUAIL RAGU WITH POLENTA

WHAT YOU NEED:

4 x quail (wild shot if possible)
4 x slices jamón
Polenta
2 x onions, finely diced
2 x carrots, finely diced
5 x garlic cloves
3.5 oz (100 g) butter
1 cup Parmesan, grated

3 cups (750 ml) passata
  (see page 212)
1/2 cup red wine
Fresh thyme, chopped
1 x red chili, diced, seeds in
Chili powder
Olive oil
Salt
Pepper

HOW TO:

Preheat your oven to 350 F (180 C).

After plucking and cleaning the bird, prepare the quail by carefully slicing the legs off the body with as much of the meat intact as possible.

Wrap each leg in the jamón. In a hot frying pan sear the legs but don't cook them for long, just give them some color.

Wrap the legs in aluminum foil, include the garlic cloves, and place in the oven for 10 minutes. When finished, open the foil and allow to cool. Set aside the quail legs and then start to remove all the meat from the birds.

In the same pan the legs were seared in, heat some olive oil and add the carrots and onions. When you have some color to them, add the passata, the roasted garlic cloves (from the aluminum packets with the legs), red wine, a sprinkle of chili powder, diced chili, thyme, and the remaining quail meat (not the legs). Let this simmer on a low heat for 15 minutes. Taste and season if required.

Cooking polenta is like cooking risotto; it takes a little love, but it's a great base that marries well with rich flavors. Bring 1 quart (1 liter) of water to boil and add 1 cup of polenta. Stir consistently for 10-15 minutes until the consistency is no longer grainy. Add your butter and Parmesan and stir for another five minutes.

Serve in bowls, with extra shaved Parmesan, olive oil, and the quail legs on top of the polenta and ragu.

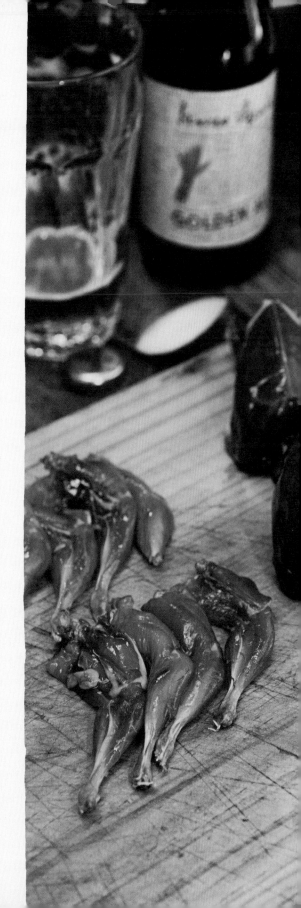

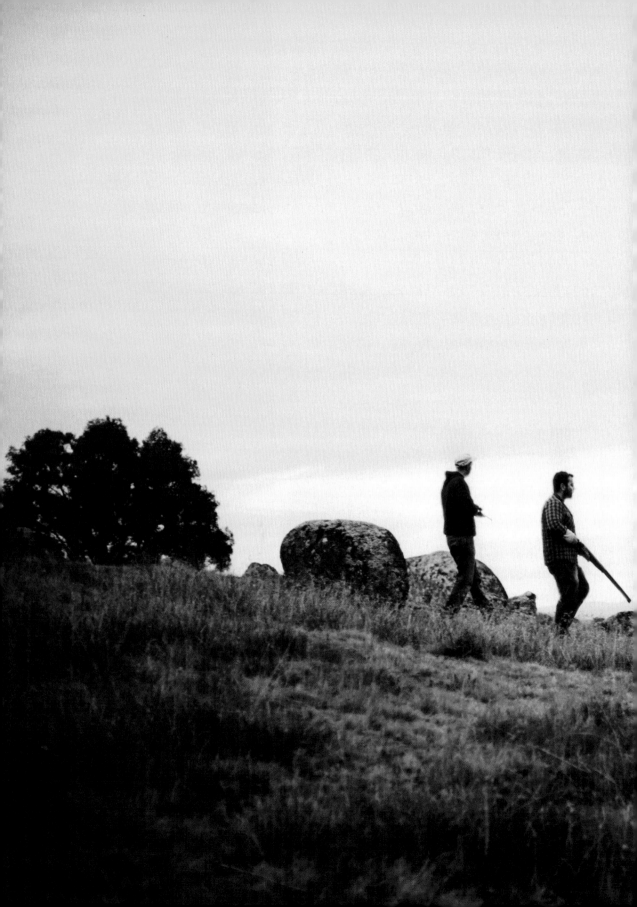

A TRUE FRIEND
LEAVES YOU WITH
MEAT FOR
YOUR FREEZER,

EVEN IF IT WAS JUST
BECAUSE HE HAD PITY
FOR YOUR BAD NIGHT.

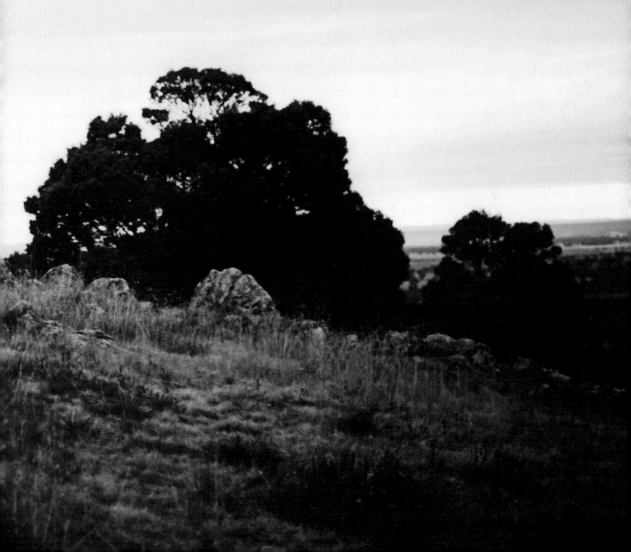

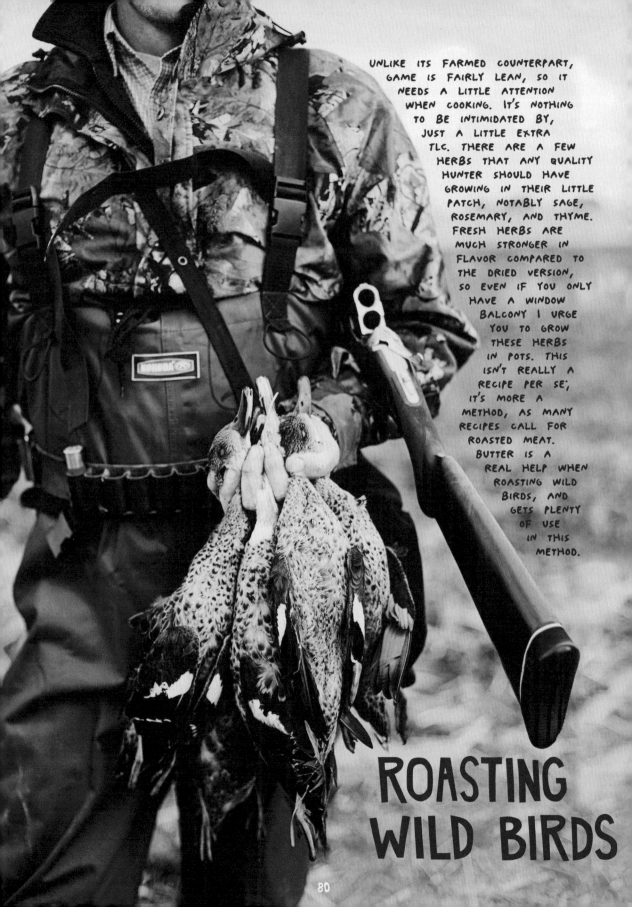

UNLIKE ITS FARMED COUNTERPART, GAME IS FAIRLY LEAN, SO IT NEEDS A LITTLE ATTENTION WHEN COOKING. IT'S NOTHING TO BE INTIMIDATED BY, JUST A LITTLE EXTRA TLC. THERE ARE A FEW HERBS THAT ANY QUALITY HUNTER SHOULD HAVE GROWING IN THEIR LITTLE PATCH, NOTABLY SAGE, ROSEMARY, AND THYME. FRESH HERBS ARE MUCH STRONGER IN FLAVOR COMPARED TO THE DRIED VERSION, SO EVEN IF YOU ONLY HAVE A WINDOW BALCONY I URGE YOU TO GROW THESE HERBS IN POTS. THIS ISN'T REALLY A RECIPE PER SE, IT'S MORE A METHOD, AS MANY RECIPES CALL FOR ROASTED MEAT. BUTTER IS A REAL HELP WHEN ROASTING WILD BIRDS, AND GETS PLENTY OF USE IN THIS METHOD.

ROASTING WILD BIRDS

WHAT YOU NEED:

1 x bird (dressed and plucked, skin on)
3.5 oz (100 g) butter
1 handful fresh sage, chopped
1 handful fresh thyme
1 sprig rosemary
Olive oil
Salt
Pepper

HOW TO:

In a bowl, mix butter with the chopped sage and thyme. Use a spoon or your fingers.

Place the bird in a baking dish, belly down. Gently peel the skin away (but not off) the back end of the bird, and then stuff in a few knobs of butter. Apply butter in this method to the neck end too, so that the topside of the bird has butter under its skin. This will help keep the bird moist during the roast.

Place the rosemary and the herbed butter mix into the rear cavity.

Using baking string, tie up the legs and back end to reduce any open holes.

Dress the bird in some olive oil, crack over some salt and pepper, and cover with aluminum foil.

Depending on your oven, roast the bird at around 350 F (180 C) for half an hour.

Feel free to check the bird as you're cooking it, as there is nothing worst than drying out a perfectly good bird and wasting good meat. I pierce the breast with a skewer and if red juice comes out it still needs some cooking time, if it's clearer then it's ready. You can also take the bird out of the oven and let it rest, it will still cook for a while especially if you leave it covered in the aluminum.

RABBIT WITH MUSTARD SAUCE

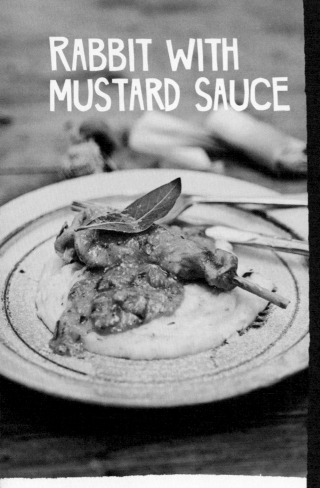

6 x rabbit legs (rear)

5.25 oz (150 g) bacon chopped

4 x onions chopped

5 x garlic cloves, chopped

2 oz (50 g) butter

2 cups (500 ml) chicken stock

1/2 cup white wine

2 tbsp of Dijon mustard

Fresh thyme, chopped

Fresh bay leaf

1/2 cup parsley, chopped

Plain flour

Olive oil

Salt

Pepper

HOW TO:

Preheat your oven to 350 F (180 C).

In a baking dish (cast iron or ceramic with lid) on a stove top, heat the butter and olive oil and brown the bacon, onion, and garlic for around 5 minutes. When done set aside.

Dust the rabbit in flour and brown in the baking dish for a few minutes on each side. Deglaze the pot with the wine on high heat. Scrape the sides of the dish into the mix as this will add to the overall flavor.

Return the bacon, onions, and garlic to the oven dish.

Add the chicken stock, thyme, and the bay leaf. Mix the ingredients well.

Pop the lid on the dish and bake for 2 hours. Flip the legs over after the first hour.

Remove the dish from the oven and check with a fork to see if the meat comes off the bones easily. If so, remove the rabbit pieces and wrap in aluminum foil and set aside.

Place the oven dish on the stove at high heat. Stir and reduce for a few minutes, until you have a thick consistency. Add the Dijon mustard and fresh, chopped parsley. Stir well.

Serve the rabbit legs on top of a dollop of mashed potatoes and drizzle over the mustard sauce.

BRAISED RABBIT RECIPES WERE A DIME A DOZEN DURING THE TOUGH POST-WAR ERA, AS RABBIT WAS PLENTIFUL AND—BETTER YET—FREE (MINUS THE COST OF A BULLET). WILD RABBIT IS VERY LEAN AND NEEDS TO BE COOKED LONGER THAN ITS FARMED EQUIVALENT BUT TASTES JUST AS GOOD!

THE LONG COOK OF THIS MEAL IS ONE OF THOSE GREAT EXCUSES TO DO NOTHING MUCH...OTHER THAN MAYBE TAKING A FEW EXTENDED SIPS FROM A FINE GLASS OF PINOT NOIR. THE MUSTARD SAUCE RABBIT IS ONE OF MY REGULAR WAYS TO COOK THIS BEAST AND IT'S ALWAYS A CROWD PLEASER. IT'S SURE TO HAVE YOUR GUESTS ASKING FOR SECONDS. REPLY BY HANDING THEM THE GUN AND TELLING THEM TO GET BUSY.

THIS RABBIT SITS NICELY ON A BED OF MASHED POTATOES, WHICH MOST PEOPLE KNOW HOW TO MAKE, SO I WON'T TELL YOU HOW TO SUCK EGGS.

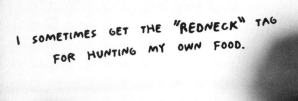

I SOMETIMES GET THE "REDNECK" TAG FOR HUNTING MY OWN FOOD.

APPARENTLY OWNING GUNS AND HUNTING BEAUTIFUL NATURAL SOURCES OF MEAT IS DEEMED BARBARIC IN THIS SYNTHETIC CULTURE.

I MUST HAVE MISSED THE MEMO.

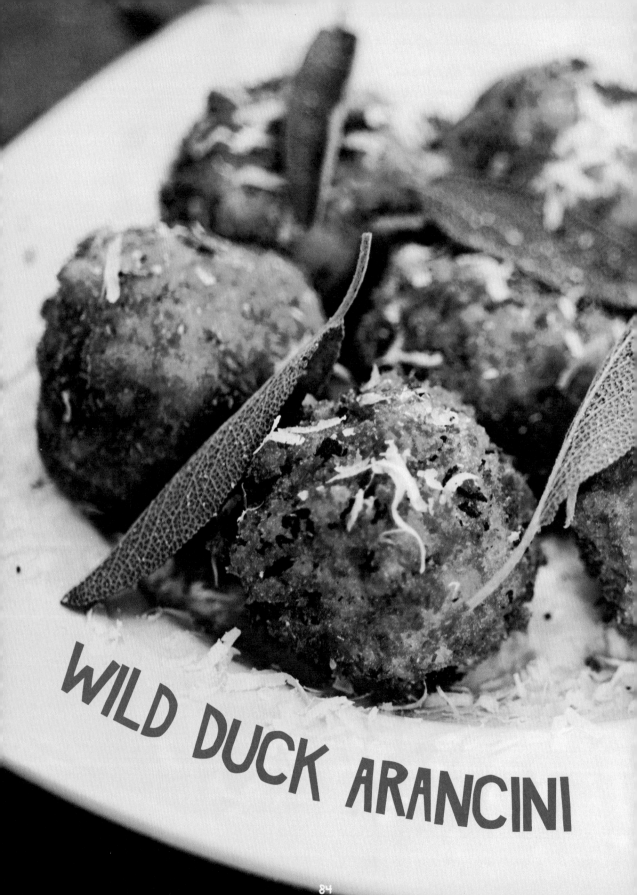

WILD DUCK ARANCINI

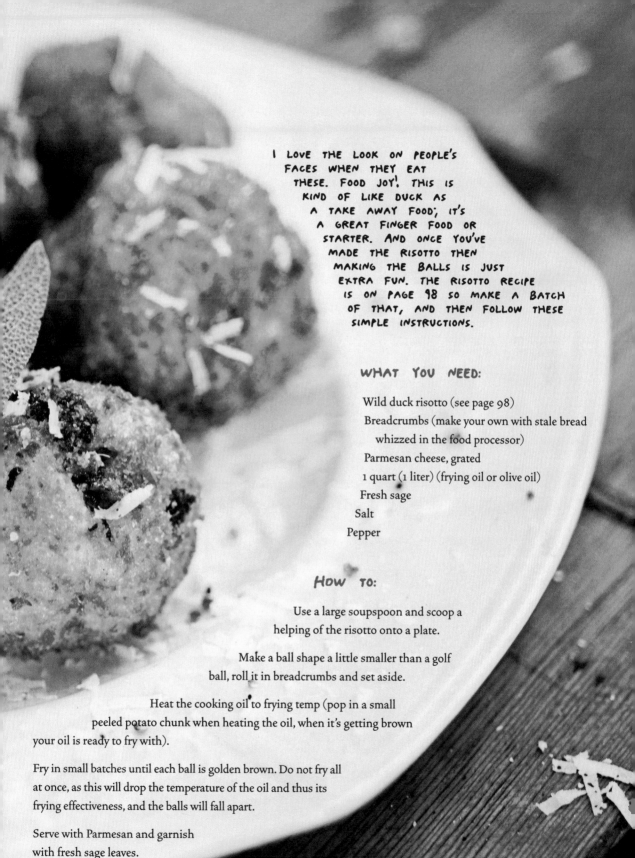

I LOVE THE LOOK ON PEOPLE'S
FACES WHEN THEY EAT
THESE. FOOD JOY! THIS IS
KIND OF LIKE DUCK AS
A TAKE AWAY FOOD; IT'S
A GREAT FINGER FOOD OR
STARTER. AND ONCE YOU'VE
MADE THE RISOTTO THEN
MAKING THE BALLS IS JUST
EXTRA FUN. THE RISOTTO RECIPE
IS ON PAGE 98 SO MAKE A BATCH
OF THAT, AND THEN FOLLOW THESE
SIMPLE INSTRUCTIONS.

WHAT YOU NEED:

Wild duck risotto (see page 98)
Breadcrumbs (make your own with stale bread
   whizzed in the food processor)
Parmesan cheese, grated
1 quart (1 liter) (frying oil or olive oil)
Fresh sage
Salt
Pepper

HOW TO:

Use a large soupspoon and scoop a
helping of the risotto onto a plate.

Make a ball shape a little smaller than a golf
ball, roll it in breadcrumbs and set aside.

Heat the cooking oil to frying temp (pop in a small
peeled potato chunk when heating the oil, when it's getting brown
your oil is ready to fry with).

Fry in small batches until each ball is golden brown. Do not fry all
at once, as this will drop the temperature of the oil and thus its
frying effectiveness, and the balls will fall apart.

Serve with Parmesan and garnish
with fresh sage leaves.

QUAIL SEASON OFTEN
COINCIDES WITH THE
MUSHROOM SEASON, SO
IT SEEMS AN OBVIOUS
MARRIAGE OF WILD FLAVORS.
QUAIL IS A LOVELY GAME
BIRD. ITS FLAVOR ISN'T TOO
STRONG OR OVERPOWERING,
SO DON'T SHY AWAY FROM
TRYING IT. AND IT'S OFTEN
WORTH TACKLING THE SMALL
FRAME TO GET AT THAT
TASTY MEAT. THIS RECIPE
WOULD WORK EQUALLY
WELL WITH OTHER SMALL,
FEATHERED GAME LIKE
PIGEON, DOVE, SMALL DUCK,
OR CHUKAR. IF YOU DON'T
HUNT THE WILD VARIETIES
YOU CAN OFTEN SOURCE
QUAIL THAT IS FARMED
OR TAP INTO A HUNTING
NETWORK.

ROAST QUAIL WITH WILD MUSHROOM + AUTUMN MASH

WHAT YOU NEED:

4 x whole quail

3.5 oz (100 g) salami, finely
   chopped

1 cup breadcrumbs

5.25 oz (150 g) wild mushrooms

1.75 oz (50 g) butter

1 handful thyme

1 handful sage

1 sprig rosemary

Olive oil

Salt

Pepper

Autumn harvest mash

1 x large potato

1/2 x butternut squash

2 x carrot

1 x onion

Butter

Olive Oil

Salt

Pepper

HOW TO:

Shoot quail.

Preheat the oven to 400 F (200 C).

Heat some butter and a splash of olive oil in a fry pan and cook the mushrooms and salami. When cooked set aside in a bowl and season.

Make the breadcrumbs using a food processor and some slices of bread a few days stale. When processed, add to the mixing bowl and mix with the salami, mushrooms, thyme, and sage. Mix all the stuffing ingredients well.

Fill the rear cavity of each bird with the stuffing mixture. Use a little knob of butter to "plug the hole."

When this is done, string tie the birds' back legs to assist closing the cavity.

Drizzle a splash of olive oil over the bird and crack over some salt and pepper.

Place in a baking tray and cover with aluminum foil. Bake for 15 minutes.

While the quail is baking, boil some water and boil all the vegetables until they can be easily pierced with a fork.

Place the cooked veg in a mixing bowl, add a generous knob of butter, a good crack of salt and pepper, and then process with a stick blender to get a creamy texture.

Spoon the mash over a plate and serve the quail on top.

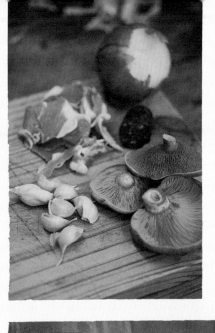

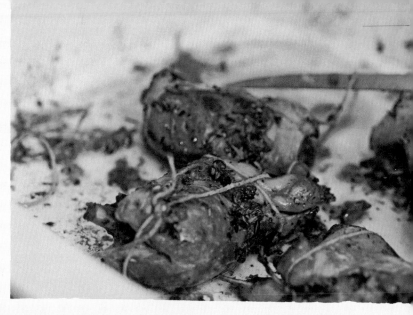

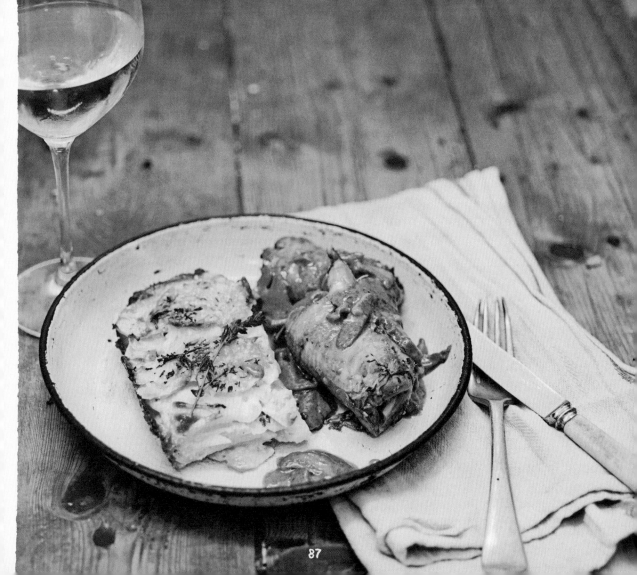

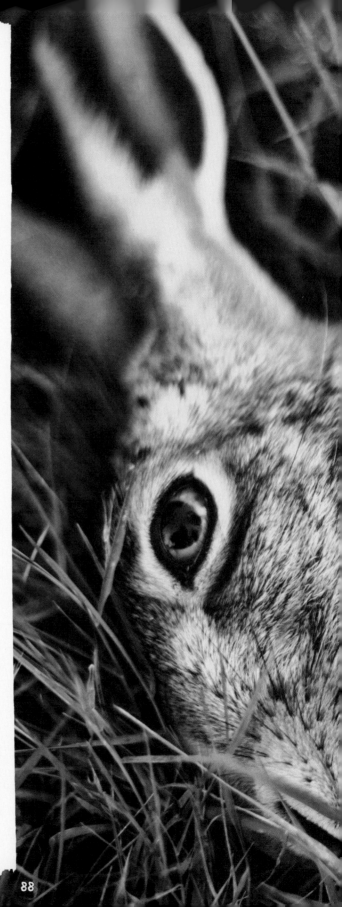

Like most things, the best advice is to start small. Hunt the small stuff like rabbit and hare; both will provide you with healthy and lean meat. With a .22 you can shoot accurately within a 30-100 yard range, a real bonus if you have yet to master the stealth of the ninja, because you won't have to creep up too close to your foe. Practice by doing. Get out there whenever you can and never give up. It sounds clichéd, but like many things it's a skill that you will only develop with plenty of practice.

Even though I live in the country, I only have a tiny backyard. To make matters worse there are no wild animals in my backyard, and trust me I've looked really hard. So, all my hunting is done on a mixture of private and public land. For the state-owned land check your local regulations, and remember safety. State-owned land is used by everyone, so when taking aim, make sure you do not shoot at anything unless you're more than certain it's not one of your kind.

For private land you'll need to utilize a mixture of charm and networking skills to garnish the landowner's approval. In Texas they have a wild boar problem, in Australia there's an invasive rabbit problem, and we all know London has the zombies. Offering to hunt game that is regarded as a pest species will help you get access to private land as landowners want to be rid of them, but may not have the time or the means to implement pest control. Do a letter drop to farms offering free vermin control, you may get one or two farmers to call you. Keep in mind that just because it's regarded as a pest, doesn't mean it won't taste good. Except zombies. They'll give you a headache.

A good, ethical shooter will aim for a clean kill shot. This is relative to the game you're hunting, but it usually means aiming straight for the head or heart. Not only will the animal be instantly dispatched, but you'll also reduce the chance of spoiling the meat. You'll understand what this means after you've shot a few animals. There is no point wasting a life with a bad shot.

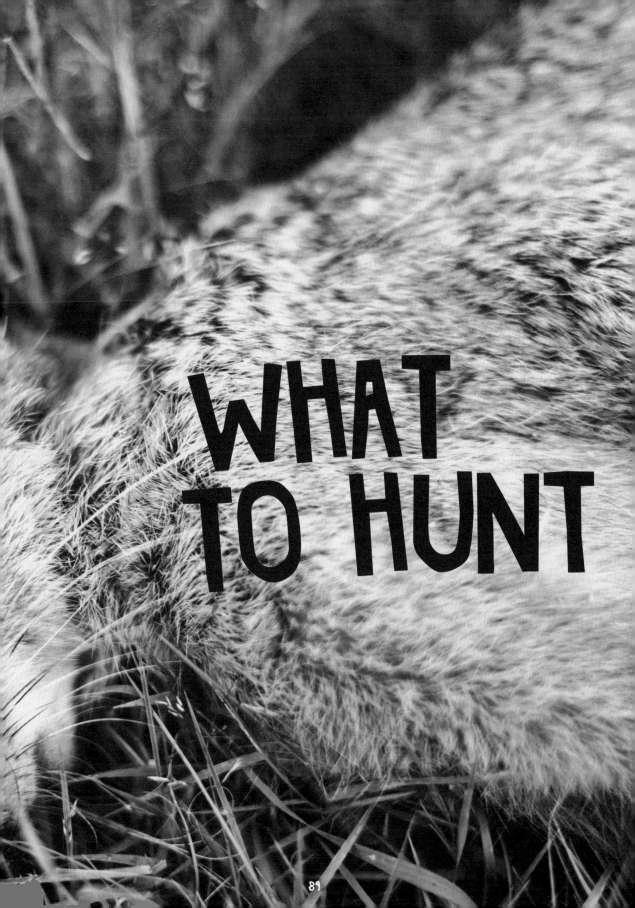

WHAT TO HUNT

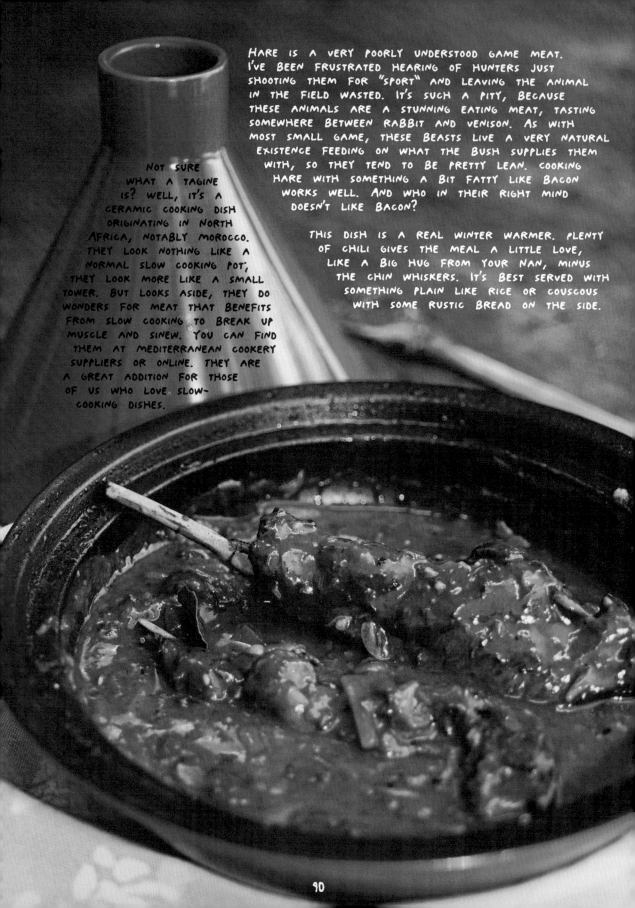

HARE IS A VERY POORLY UNDERSTOOD GAME MEAT. I'VE BEEN FRUSTRATED HEARING OF HUNTERS JUST SHOOTING THEM FOR "SPORT" AND LEAVING THE ANIMAL IN THE FIELD WASTED. IT'S SUCH A PITY, BECAUSE THESE ANIMALS ARE A STUNNING EATING MEAT, TASTING SOMEWHERE BETWEEN RABBIT AND VENISON. AS WITH MOST SMALL GAME, THESE BEASTS LIVE A VERY NATURAL EXISTENCE FEEDING ON WHAT THE BUSH SUPPLIES THEM WITH, SO THEY TEND TO BE PRETTY LEAN. COOKING HARE WITH SOMETHING A BIT FATTY LIKE BACON WORKS WELL. AND WHO IN THEIR RIGHT MIND DOESN'T LIKE BACON?

NOT SURE WHAT A TAGINE IS? WELL, IT'S A CERAMIC COOKING DISH ORIGINATING IN NORTH AFRICA, NOTABLY MOROCCO. THEY LOOK NOTHING LIKE A NORMAL SLOW COOKING POT; THEY LOOK MORE LIKE A SMALL TOWER. BUT LOOKS ASIDE, THEY DO WONDERS FOR MEAT THAT BENEFITS FROM SLOW COOKING TO BREAK UP MUSCLE AND SINEW. YOU CAN FIND THEM AT MEDITERRANEAN COOKERY SUPPLIERS OR ONLINE. THEY ARE A GREAT ADDITION FOR THOSE OF US WHO LOVE SLOW-COOKING DISHES.

THIS DISH IS A REAL WINTER WARMER. PLENTY OF CHILI GIVES THE MEAL A LITTLE LOVE, LIKE A BIG HUG FROM YOUR NAN, MINUS THE CHIN WHISKERS. IT'S BEST SERVED WITH SOMETHING PLAIN LIKE RICE OR COUSCOUS WITH SOME RUSTIC BREAD ON THE SIDE.

HARE TAGINE

WHAT YOU NEED:

4 x hare, back legs

3.5 oz (100gm) bacon

2 x onions

2 x carrots

5 x cloves, garlic

1 tbsp juniper berries, crushed

1 x large dried chili, chopped

2 cups beef stock

1 x cup red wine

1/2 cup Fino sherry

2 x tsp paprika

2 x fresh bay leaf

1 x chorizo sausage

Olive oil

Salt

Pepper

HOW TO:

Chop up your garlic, onions, and carrots. Set aside in a bowl.

Chop up the chorizo and bacon. Set aside in a bowl.

Heat glug of olive oil in the tagine.

In the tagine, cook the sausage and bacon on high heat for at least 5 minutes, or until soft. Then remove and set aside.

In the tagine, cook the garlic, onion, and carrots on medium heat for at least 5 minutes. Then remove and set aside.

On high heat, brown the hare pieces on each side for a few minutes. Don't overcook them! You just want to sear them.

Return everything (the veggies, the chopped meat, and the hare) to the tagine. Mix well.

Add the wine, sherry, stock, bay leaf, paprika, and chopped chili. Mix well, making sure all the flavors amalgamate.

Cook on low heat in the tagine with the lid on for 2 – 5 hours, or until meat falls off the bone.

Remove the legs and let stand covered in tin foil.

With the lid removed from the tagine, turn the heat up high and reduce the sauce for 5 minutes, stirring well. Season with S&P.

Serve the legs on a bed of couscous or steamed rice, drizzle with a generous serve of the sauce and a sprinkle of chopped parsley.

NB: If you don't have Fino sherry, then use dry sherry.

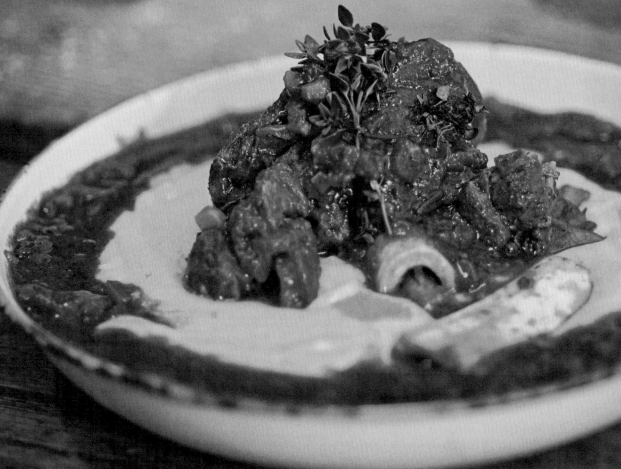

It's a lot of work hunting deer. It requires patience, skill, and gritty determination. Luckily for us, we have some deer hunter friends that we trade with. And if that option isn't available, we're blessed with a local venison farm. We often prefer the cheaper cuts of meat, for one obvious reason— they're cheaper! But they also present more interesting flavors, even if they take a little longer to cook. This meal is a hearty autumn/winter treat that we serve on polenta, and devour by the warmth of the fireplace with a nice glass or two of red.

VENISON OSSOBUCO

WHAT YOU NEED:

6 x venison ossobuco

Polenta

2 x onions, chopped

2 x carrots, chopped

2 x sticks celery, chopped

24 oz (700 ml) passata (see page 212)

2 cups venison stock (or chicken)

1 cup Fino sherry

Small bunch fresh parsley

1 tsp juniper berries

2 fresh bay leaves

1 sprig rosemary

Flour

Oilve Oil

Salt

Pepper

HOW TO:

Heat an oven-safe cooking pot on the stovetop and add a glug of olive oil.

Add the diced carrots, onion, and celery, while stirring often for 10-15 minutes. When cooked, remove the veggies and set aside.

Lightly flour each piece of meat and in the same cooking pot brown the venison on all sides for a few minutes. When done, return the vegetables to the pot.

With the dish still on the heat, pour in the Fino sherry and cook for a few minutes stirring well.

Now add the passata, juniper berries, parsley, bay leaves, rosemary, and stock and season.

Place the lid on and cook in the oven on a medium heat 325 F (160 C) for at least 1.5 hours, or until the meat is tender.

Remove the cooked meat from the pot and set aside, covered with aluminum foil.

Push the remaining contents in the pot through a sieve, and return this sauce to the pot along with the meat. Keep the baking dish in the oven at a warming temp, but not cooking.

Cook the polenta as per packet instructions. Best to start this process 30 minutes prior to when the meat will finish cooking.

Serve the polenta in a bowl with the meat on top, drizzled with the rich sauce.

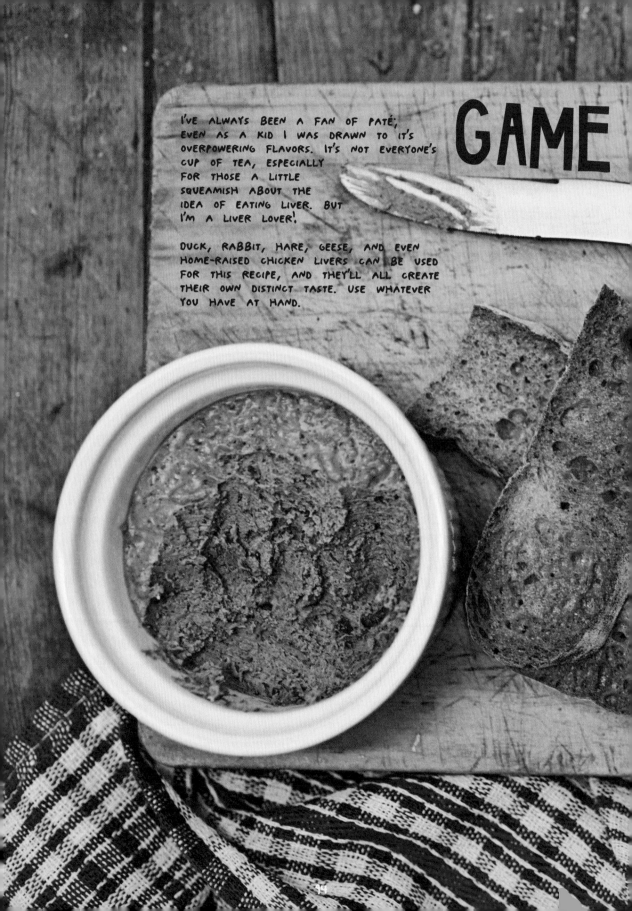

I'VE ALWAYS BEEN A FAN OF PATÉ;
EVEN AS A KID I WAS DRAWN TO IT'S
OVERPOWERING FLAVORS. IT'S NOT EVERYONE'S
CUP OF TEA, ESPECIALLY
FOR THOSE A LITTLE
SQUEAMISH ABOUT THE
IDEA OF EATING LIVER. BUT
I'M A LIVER LOVER!

DUCK, RABBIT, HARE, GEESE, AND EVEN
HOME-RAISED CHICKEN LIVERS CAN BE USED
FOR THIS RECIPE, AND THEY'LL ALL CREATE
THEIR OWN DISTINCT TASTE. USE WHATEVER
YOU HAVE AT HAND.

GAME

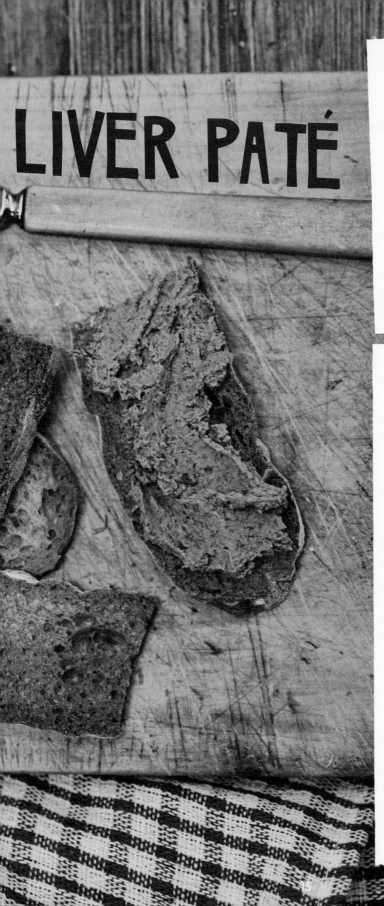

LIVER PATÉ

WHAT YOU NEED:

6–8 livers

4 rashers smoky bacon (or
   pancetta)

1 x onion, chopped

3.5 oz (100 g) butter (or equivalent to the weight of the livers)

1/2 cup (100 ml) pouring cream

Brandy

Fresh thyme, finely chopped

Fresh sage, finely chopped

Olive oil

Salt

Pepper

HOW TO:

Heat some olive oil in a frying pan
and brown your onions and bacon
(6 minutes). Set aside.

Chop the livers into chunks and add
to the same pan, cooking them for
about 10 minutes, turning regularly.
Remove from the heat and set aside
with the bacon and onions.

Deglaze the pan with the brandy.
Add a knob of butter and the finely
chopped fresh thyme and sage.
Now return the bacon, livers, and
onions to the pan for a quick few
minutes, mixing well.

Transfer all cooked ingredients
into a food processor and give it a
good mix until the texture is very
fine. Add butter in chunks, and
when completely mixed remove the
lid and stir in the cream. Season
to taste.

Pour into ramekins and refrigerate
overnight.

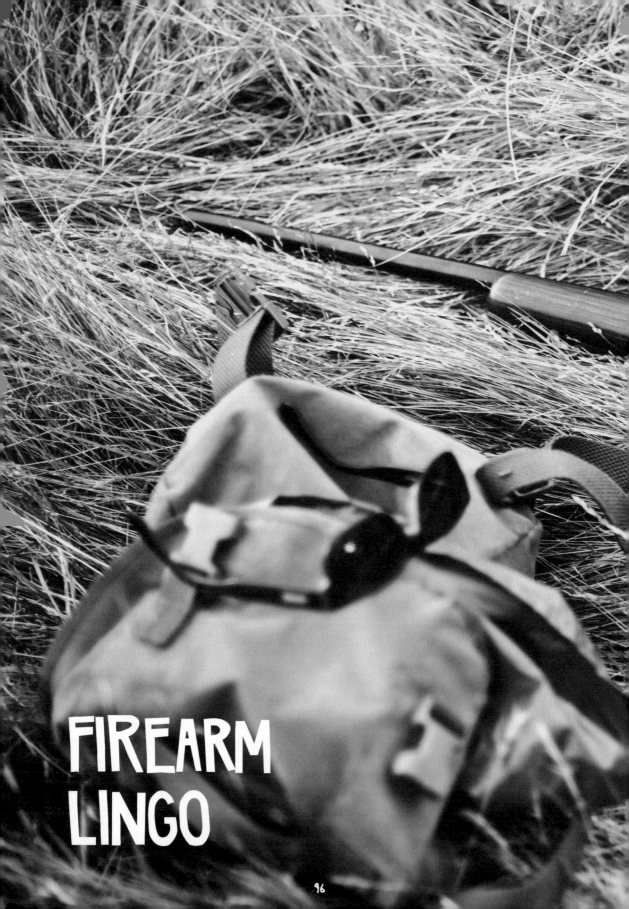

FIREARM
LINGO

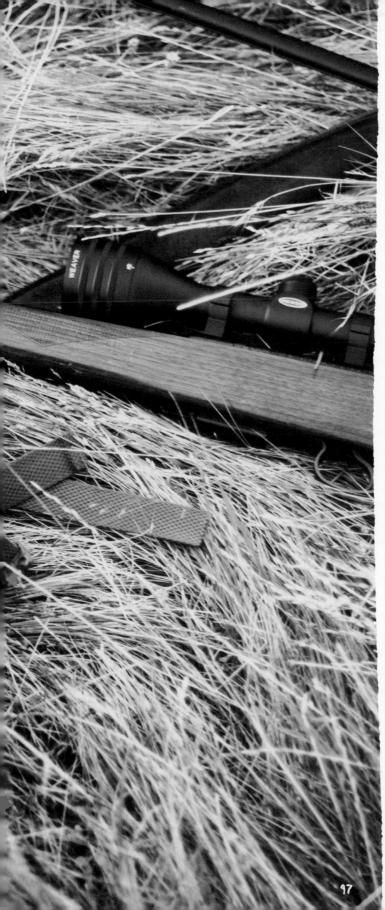

Your first time at the shooting range or hunting club, you may find that the fellows there are speaking a foreign language. Before you arrive it will be helpful to have an understanding of some basic firearm terminology.

ACTION: Generally speaking this refers to how the firing mechanism works. There are two main types, lever action and bolt action. Lever action is John-Wayne, cowboy-style. Bolt action is an elephant hunter in Africa. Both do the same job, which is firing a projectile. The difference is safety. A bolt action is considered a safer option because the action can be totally removed, thus rendering the rifle inoperable. Another safety aspect of a bolt action is that the shooter can easily see a round loaded in the chamber (a bullet ready, and seated in the firing position). In most lever actions the rounds are stored in a secondary barrel under the firing barrel and it's impossible to see whether there are live rounds in the chamber, so you'll need to keep count. I'm not so good at counting, thus my preference for the bolt action.

CALIBER: The size of the diameter of the barrel, which is determined by the size of the projectile.

CENTERFIRE: The action hits the casing in the centre (usually applies to large caliber rifles).

PROJECTILE: The pointy bit of the bullet.

RIMFIRE: The action hits the outside rim at the back of the casing (usually applies to small caliber rifles).

A ROUND: An individual bullet.

A SHELL: A shotgun casing.

WILD DUCK RISOTTO

THIS IS A PERFECT COOL WEATHER MEAL THAT I RECKON IS THE PERFECT PEASANT FOOD. IT WILL BRING JOY TO ALL THOSE WHO DEVOUR IT. OFTEN PEOPLE SEEM TO BE SCARED OFF BY THE THOUGHT OF ATTEMPTING TO COOK RISOTTO, BUT HONESTLY IT'S JUST A RICE STEW WITH A LOT OF STIRRING. EVEN MY DAD COULD MAKE THIS. ACTUALLY, ON SECOND THOUGHT, DAD, PLEASE DON'T TRY IT—STICK TO YOUR "COOKING" ON THE BBQ.

YOU CAN USE EITHER WILD DUCK OR FARMED DUCK. YOU CAN USE WILD MUSHROOMS OR YOU CAN USE STORE BOUGHT. BUT IF YOU TRULY WANT TO EAT WITH THE SEASONS THEN THIS WOULD BE AN AUTUMN DISH, WHEN WILD MUSHROOMS ARE PLENTIFUL.

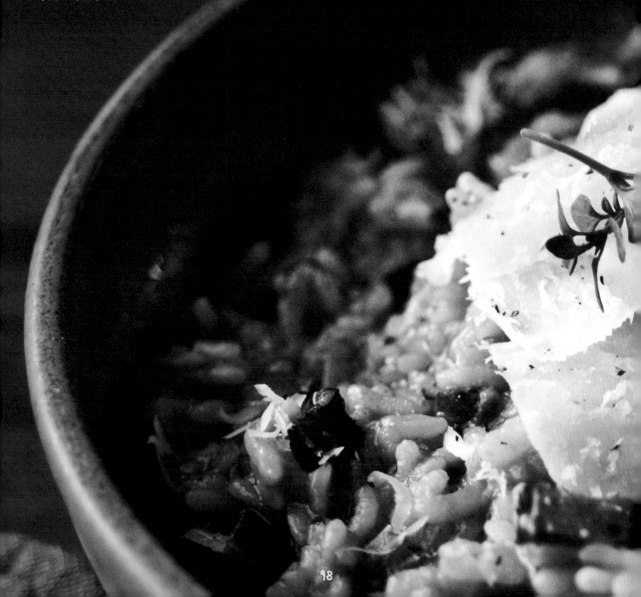

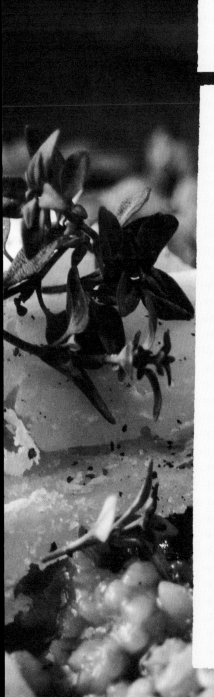

The meat from one roast duck (see page 80 for roasting wild duck)

1 lb (500 g) Arborio rice

2 cups mushrooms

2 stalks celery, diced

1 x onion, diced

5 x cloves garlic

1/2 gallon (2 liters) chicken stock

1 cup red wine

1.75 oz (50 g) butter

2 cups Parmesan, grated

Fresh thyme, finely chopped

Fresh sage, finely chopped

Olive oil

Salt

Pepper

HOW TO:

Pour your stock into a saucepan and heat on medium/low until it's warmed, but not boiling.

In a separate large saucepan, heat olive oil on a medium heat. Add your onions, garlic, and celery and cook until soft (around 8 minutes).

Add the Arborio rice and turn up to high heat, while stirring with vigor. You will see the rice lose that white color and become almost clear. This takes at least 5 minutes. Add the wine and cook out completely.

Now start adding a ladle of warmed stock, one at a time, and stir through the rice until it's been absorbed and the liquid cooked out. Best to do this on a medium to hot heat.

Repeat this process over and over again while sneaking a glass or two of the cooking wine and chatting with friends.

Order someone to finely chop the mushrooms and duck meat into yummy little pieces.

Tell them they're doing it wrong, whilst stirring and adding stock.

This will last about half an hour, now add the duck, mushrooms, and herbs. Turn the heat down and stir to get all the flavors introduced to each other. Mushrooms meet sage, sage meet duck. Formal introductions are optional. Best not to let people see you talking to your food.

Turn the heat off and add the Parmesan cheese and butter and pop the lid on for a few minutes. Once melted, stir, and season to taste. Serve topped with a little glug of good quality virgin olive oil.

ROAST DUCK RAGU PASTA BAKE

WHAT YOU NEED:

Meat from a roast wild duck, roughly chopped
3 x large pork sausages, chopped
1 lb (500 g) pasta (anything short like penne, bows, or tubes)
3 x carrots, diced
2 x celery sticks, diced
1 x onion, diced
5 x cloves garlic, diced
1 x fresh chili
1-2 cups mozzarella, grated
Parmesan, grated
24 oz passata (see page 212)
2 cups water
1 tbsp chili oil (see page 207)
2 sprigs fresh rosemary, finely chopped
1 bunch fresh sage, finely chopped
Olive oil
Salt
Pepper

HOW TO:

Roast the duck (p 80). Remember that it's wild and don't overcook it. To retain moisture you can roast it covered in aluminum foil. Once roasted allow it to cool enough to handle and remove and roughly chop the meat.

In a large saucepan, heat a glug of olive oil. Brown the onion, garlic, celery, and carrots. When done, remove and set aside.

In the same saucepan, cook the sausage until seared well. When done, return the cooked the veg to the pan, add the roasted duck meat and stir well.

Add the passata, chili oil, chopped chili, and the herbs.

Simmer on a low heat for an hour. As it reduces add the extra water.

After an hour, cook the pasta al dente.

In a large baking dish, mix the pasta and the ragu sauce well, spreading it out in the dish evenly.

Cover the top of the pasta with shredded mozzarella and grate some Parmesan over that.

Bake for 20 minutes at 400 F (200 C) until the cheese is crisp.

Serve to hungry guests.

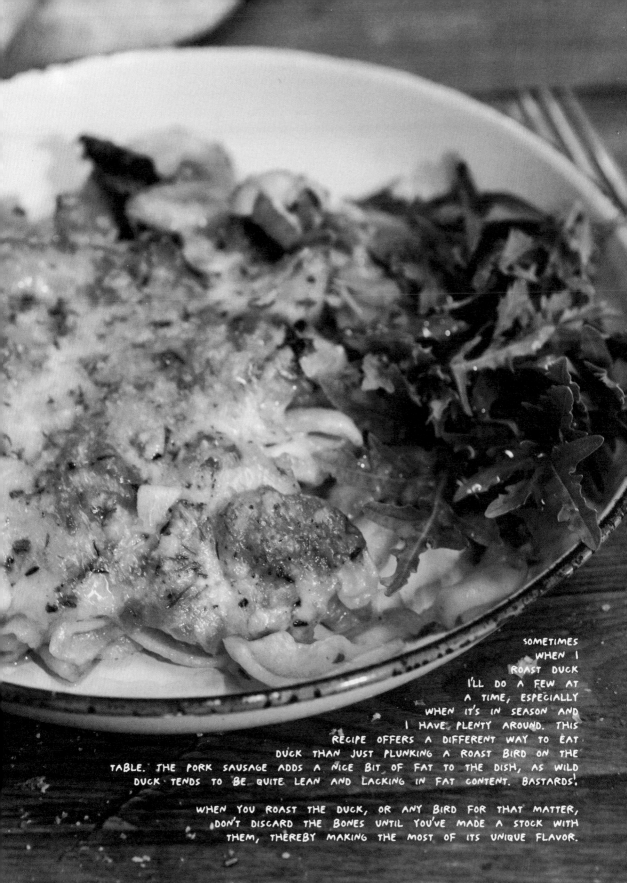

SOMETIMES
WHEN I
ROAST DUCK
I'LL DO A FEW AT
A TIME, ESPECIALLY
WHEN IT'S IN SEASON AND
I HAVE PLENTY AROUND. THIS
RECIPE OFFERS A DIFFERENT WAY TO EAT
DUCK THAN JUST PLUNKING A ROAST BIRD ON THE
TABLE. THE PORK SAUSAGE ADDS A NICE BIT OF FAT TO THE DISH, AS WILD
DUCK TENDS TO BE QUITE LEAN AND LACKING IN FAT CONTENT. BASTARDS!

WHEN YOU ROAST THE DUCK, OR ANY BIRD FOR THAT MATTER,
DON'T DISCARD THE BONES UNTIL YOU'VE MADE A STOCK WITH
THEM, THEREBY MAKING THE MOST OF ITS UNIQUE FLAVOR.

(SORRY ABOUT THE PIC OF THE RABBIT, BUT HE LIVED A HAPPY LIFE, MUCH BETTER THAN MANY FARMED MEATS THAT YOU CAN PICK UP AT THE SUPERMARKET AND NOT THINK TWICE ABOUT.)

SKINNING + PREPARING A RABBIT

So you've shot, snagged or jumped on a wild rabbit... well done! Now, to get it cleaned up. It's best to do it as soon as you have access to a clean working area, running water, and a fridge or freezer unless you plan on cooking it straight away.

First, grab a sharp hunting knife. Pinch the fur on the chest between the two front paws. Make an incision and then prise the fur and skin off the belly. I tend to cut down along the fur as I'm pulling it away from the skin. I cut from the chest to the tail.

Now you'll see the pink meat of the belly, make a cut at the top of the belly down towards the bum, while making sure not to pierce any of the internal organs.

When you've got an open cut the length of the belly, place your hand in and pull out all the organs. Keep the livers if you want to make pate!

Discard the guts making sure not to cut into them, as the smell will put you off ever attempting this task again.

Now you can really start to peel the fur off the meat. There are a few different techniques; I tend to start from the bum and peel off towards the head. Then I'll use a large meat cleaver to chop off the feet and head. There is a lot of sinew that is attached to the outside of the meat and also extra single hairs, make sure you take your time to remove as much of this as possible. Clean your beast!

Give the body a good rinse under cold, running water then place it in a large pot of cold, salted water overnight. This will remove a little bit of the gamey flavor and it tends to whiten the meat a little. It's now ready to cook or freeze.

VINDALOO HARE

On the surface, one would think that vindaloo is just another Indian curry, but its origins are actually Portuguese. No matter where it comes from, it's a very delicious hot dish that will warm your pants off on a cold night.

WHAT YOU NEED:

2 x hare, quartered and chopped
    into chunks
1 tin diced tomatoes
1 x carrot
1 x onion
2 x cloves garlic
1.75 oz (50 g) butter
1 x cup natural yogurt
1 x cup of beef stock
3 tbsp vindaloo paste
1 bunch fresh coriander
Olive oil

HOW TO:

Heat butter and olive oil in a large slow-cooking pot (with lid) and brown the hare for a few minutes on each side then set aside.

In the same pot heat olive oil and brown the onion, garlic, and carrots until soft.

Return the hare pieces to the pot, adding the vindaloo paste, tomatoes, and beef stock. Stir all the ingredients well.

Pop the lid on and gently simmer on low heat for 1.5 hours checking after the first 40 minutes. Stir hare pieces around and check the dish isn't drying out or simmering too hot.

Remove the lid and simmer for a further 10 minutes.

Mix the coriander and yogurt and serve the hare with this sauce on a bed of steamed jasmine rice, and a cold glass of beer, maybe Asahi.

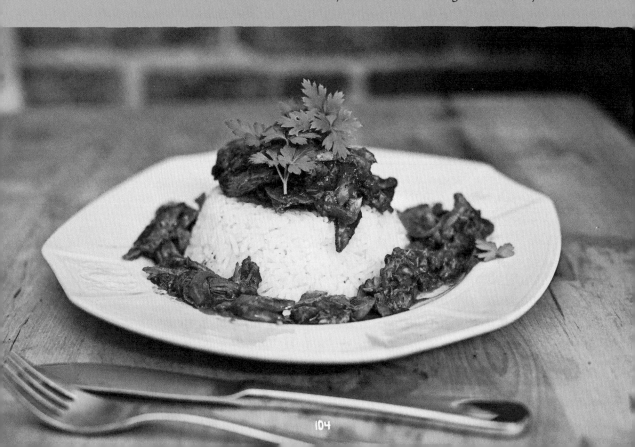

FINGER LICKIN' RABBIT

A FRIEND SHARED THIS
RECIPE WITH ME SOME
TIME BACK. IT'S ACTUALLY
A RECIPE THAT HIS MUM
MAKES FOR RABBIT. IT'S
A LITTLE RIPPER! IT'S A
BIT EVIL, BEING DEEP-
FRIED, BUT THE CRUNCH
OF THE CRISPY, FRIED
BREAD CRUMBS, AND THE
SUCCULENT MEAT, FINISHED
OFF WITH A DIP IN AIOLI
SAUCE—JUST DIVINE! IT'S
NOT SOMETHING YOU'D COOK
EVERY DAY BUT IT'S A
GREAT TREAT AND ALSO
A GOOD ONE TO FEED
KIDS. THEY LOVE IT. YOU
CAN SPICE IT UP WITH
WHATEVER SEASONING YOU
LIKE. I'VE CHANGED IT A
LITTLE FROM THE ORIGINAL
RECIPE TO SUIT MY TASTES,
SO GO AHEAD AND PUT
YOUR OWN STAMP ON IT,
BUT I ADVISE AGAINST
USING ACTUAL STAMPS.
THEY DON'T TASTE GOOD.

IF YOU'RE BUYING RABBIT,
BEST TO GET YOUNG
RABBIT. IF YOU'RE HUNTING
RABBIT, POLITELY INQUIRE
AS TO THEIR AGE PRIOR TO
SHOOTING THEM.

WHAT YOU NEED:

1-2 x rabbit, quartered and cut into chunks
6 x eggs
1 tbsp chicken stock powder
1 tbsp chicken salt
2 tsp garlic powder
2 tsp season-all
1 tsp sweet paprika
1 tbsp dried chili flakes
2 cups flour
2 cups bread crumbs
Olive oil
Salt
Pepper

HOW TO:

Cut the rabbit into small pieces.

Beat the eggs in a bowl.

Place flour, salt, pepper, garlic powder, season-all, chicken stock powder, and chicken salt into a plastic bag. Shake bag well, transfer into large mixing bowl.

Heat up olive oil in a frying pan, approx 1 inch deep.

Dip rabbit into egg.

Dip rabbit into flour mixture.

Dip rabbit into egg.

Dip rabbit into breadcrumbs.

Fry slowly until golden brown (don't have the oil too hot as you will cook the outside but not the inside...savvy!!)

Then eat and enjoy!

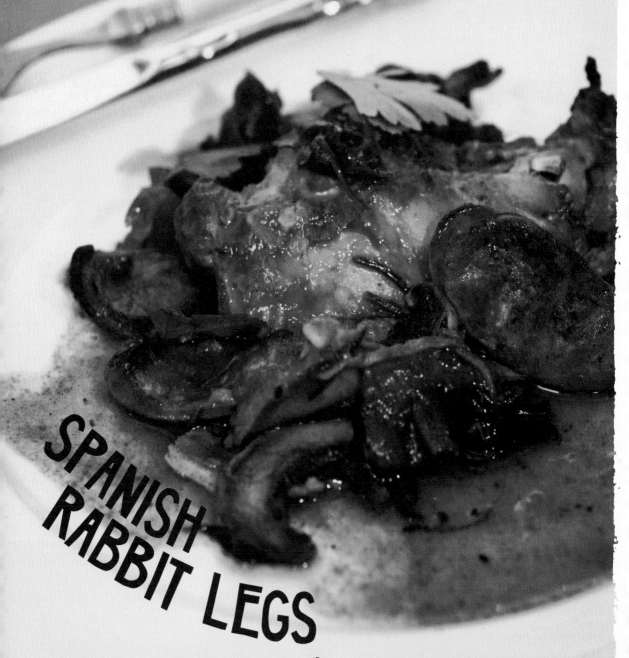

THIS MEAL HAS SOME INFLUENCES FROM THE CATALONIA REGION OF NORTHEAST SPAIN, NOTABLY THE USE OF CINNAMON. TO ALL THE FOODIES OUT THERE, DON'T BE GETTING ALL ANTSY BECAUSE I'M NOT CLAIMING IT'S A PURIST'S CATALAN MEAL. I DEFINITELY DON'T WANT TO BE ONE TO PISS OF A CATALAN! MUCHO RESPETO! IN ANY CASE THIS IS ONE OF MY FAVORITE WAYS TO DEVOUR THE LEGS OF A RABBIT OR TWO! WHEN THE MEAT FALLS OFF THE BONE, WITH A MOUTHFUL OF CHORIZO AND PROSCIUTTO, ALL COVERED IN THAT SHERRY AND TOMATO INFUSED SAUCE...HEAVENLY!

SPANISH RABBIT LEGS

WHAT YOU NEED:

Rabbit legs from two rabbits. That's 8 legs in all. (I'm really good at maths)

2 x chorizo sausages, chopped

5 slices prosciutto, shredded

5 x large wild mushrooms, chopped

6 x cloves garlic

24 oz (700 ml) passata (see page 212)

1 cup Spanish Fino sherry (or dry white wine)

2 x quills cinnamon

3 x bay leaves

1 sprig fresh rosemary

1 heaped tbsp fresh thyme

Plain flour

Olive oil

Salt

Pepper

HOW TO:

Preheat oven to 325 F (160 C) conventional heat, not convection.

Heat a glug of olive oil in a large frying pan on high heat.

Dust the rabbit in flour and brown all sides. Once done, set aside in a baking dish.

In the same pan, separately cook the chorizo, then the mushrooms. The chorizo just needs a quick little fry and the mushrooms should be cooked until they have reduced in size. When done, transfer into the baking dish with the browned rabbit.

Add the passata, cinnamon quills, garlic, herbs, bay leaf, and sherry. Mix up all the ingredients and season. Lay the shredded prosciutto over the top.

Cook covered for 2 hours. After the first hour of cooking check fluid levels and top off with hot water if necessary.

During the second hour check to see if the meat is tenderly falling from the bone.

Serve each plate with a few legs and spoon over the sauce from the baking dish.

Serve with homemade bread and a glass of Spanish vino.

USE THE RIGHT TOOL

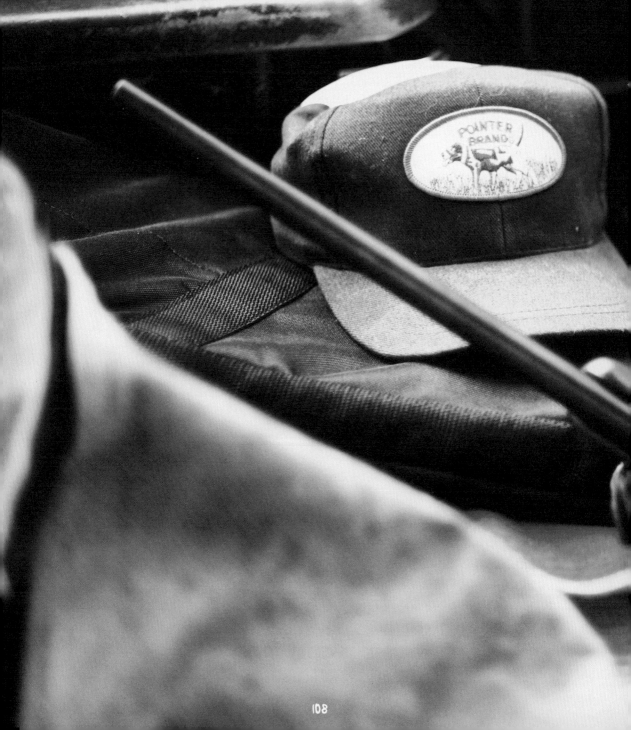

If you're hunting feathered game, then a shotgun is your gun of choice as it shoots out tiny lead/steel shots that look like ball bearings. These disperse in a spray pattern that covers more space than a single projectile, making it a practical choice for small, fast, flying game that isn't polite enough to stay still long enough for you to get a clean shot.

Furred, small game like rabbit, hare, and even wild goat can all be hunted with a .22 or a .17 caliber rifle. These are lightweight guns that can easily be carried on long hikes. But their size is not so important; it's what they do to your game that's more relevant. They can make a clean kill without too much mess. If you used a larger caliber you'd blast a big hole in the animal, and most likely spoil the meat, rendering the whole process pointless. You can use a shotgun for furred game, but you'll have to pick out the shot prior to eating—or from the bottom of your toilet bowl—hence my preference for a small caliber rifle.

If you're hunting the big stuff—deer, moose, kangaroo, or giant mutant octopus—then a larger caliber, centerfire is the way to go, perhaps a .308 or larger.

This is just basic information to help you along. Remember, your best friend in this business is the bloke behind the counter at your local gun shop. Pick their brains (not literally, that is unless you're a zombie, in which case bon appétit). They have a wealth of knowledge and will give you lots of advice.

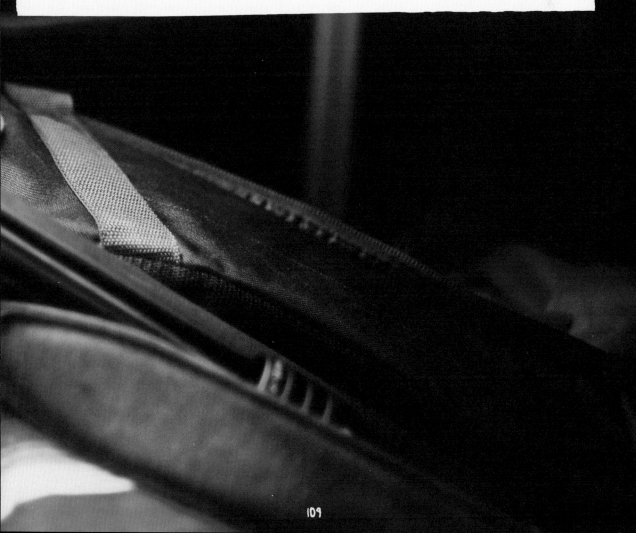

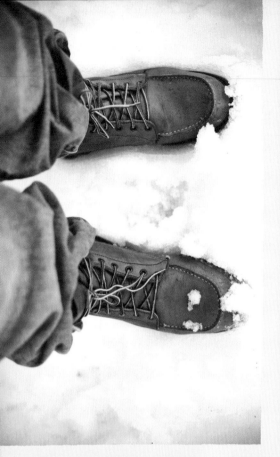

LEATHER LACE-UP BOOTS

FEET: YOU KNOW, THE THINGS THAT TAKE YOU EVERYWHERE. THEY CARRY US THROUGH OUR WHOLE LIVES, SO THEY SHOULD BE ADORNED WITH SOMETHING PRACTICAL AND FIT FOR THAT PURPOSE. I'M YET TO FIND ANYTHING THAT BEATS AMERICAN-MADE HUNTING/WORK BOOTS. THE CRAFTSMANSHIP, PRACTICALITY, AND DURABILITY ARE UNDENIABLY SUPERIOR TO ANYTHING ELSE I'VE SEEN. IF YOU TREAT THEM WITH RESPECT, THEY'LL LAST FOREVER. POLISH THEM WITH A LEATHER RUB LIKE DUBBIN OR HONEY WAX. DO THIS EVERY FEW MONTHS TO SOFTEN THE LEATHER AND IMPROVE WATERPROOFING. THESE BOOTS ARE SUITED TO WINTER HUNTING AND HIKING AND IN THE SUMMER THEY'LL KEEP YOUR FEET DRY AND GIVE YOU SOME SNAKE PROTECTION. GET SOMETHING ALONG THE LINES OF AN L.L. BEAN BOOT OR A RED WING LACE-UP. REMEMBER, A PAIR OF HANDMADE LEATHER BOOTS THAT ARE LOOKED AFTER WILL LAST YOU A GOOD MANY YEARS. THEY'RE USUALLY BUILT TO LAST.

THE BLOOD BAG

THIS IS A HESSIAN BAG THAT I'VE LINED WITH PLASTIC TO STOP BLOOD FROM GETTING EVERYWHERE. IT'S THE BAG I SLING OVER MY SHOULDER WHEN I'M HUNTING SMALL FURRED GAME. IT'S A MUST AND I ALWAYS CARRY IT IN THE JEEP.

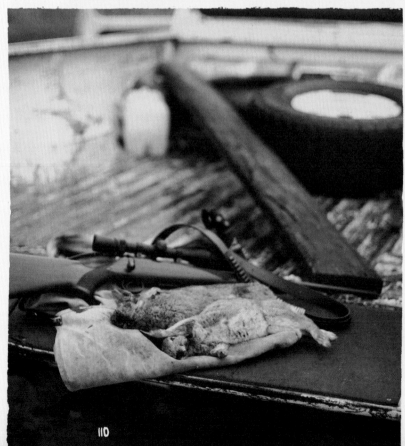

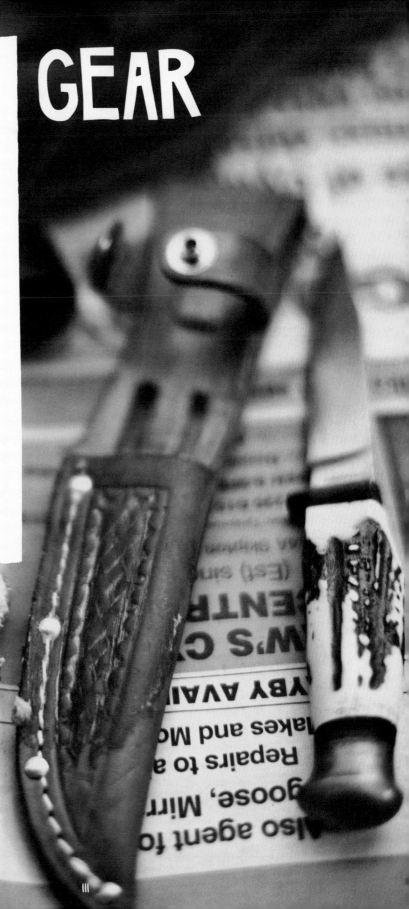

GEAR

A DECENT POCKET KNIFE/ LEATHERMAN/MULTI-TOOL:

DON'T SKIMP ON THIS.
STICK WITH THE CLASSICS,
AND PLEASE DON'T BE
CONVINCED TO BUY ONE
OF THOSE MASSIVE
LEATHERMANS WITH FORTY
TOOLS IN ONE. THE BASIC
ONE WILL DO ALMOST
ANYTHING YOU NEED,
FROM SKINNING A RABBIT
TO CUTTING FRESH SAGE.

JACKET:

UNLESS YOU LIVE IN THE
TROPICS YOU WILL GET
ALL FOUR SEASONS. THE
AMOUNT OF TIMES A
DECENT JACKET HAS SAVED
MY SANITY OUT IN THE
BUSH OR THE GARDEN
IS RECORD BREAKING.
REALLY I SHOULD JUST
GIVE UP AND GO INSIDE
BUT THERE ARE THINGS
THAT NEED TO BE DONE,
AND A DECENT LINED
JACKET (WITH AN ELEMENT
OF WATERPROOFING) IS
PRICELESS.

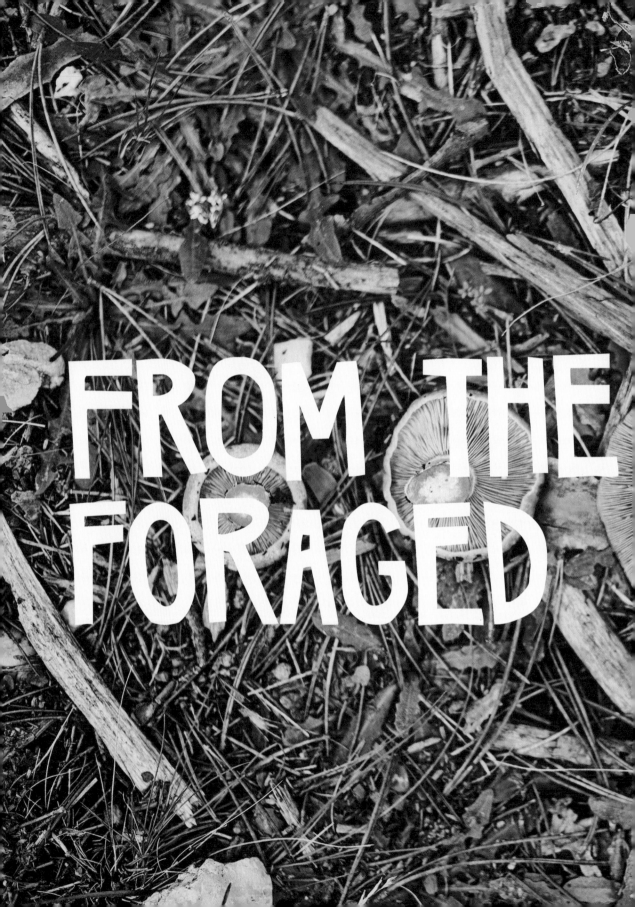

FROM THE
FORAGED

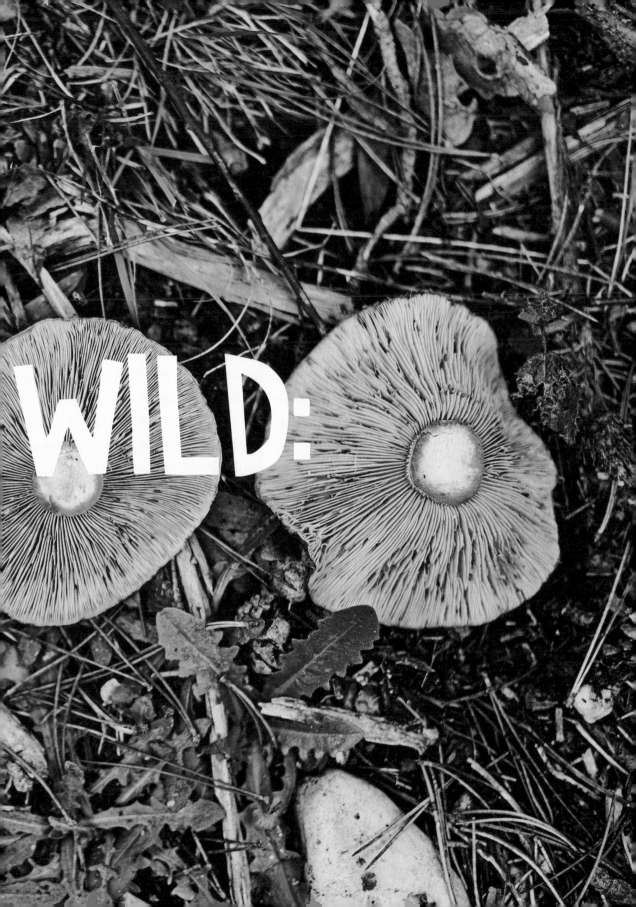

I grew up on a small farm where we raised a handful of cattle and tended a vegetable plot and fruit orchard. We had plenty of fresh food, thanks to my mother's dream of living self-sufficiently. We also enjoyed the fruits that nature provided, with little effort required on our behalf other than collecting it.

Field mushroom season was always a joy. Our paddocks would start to provide one, then two patches, and then so many patches of mushrooms we had to take buckets to harvest them. We had mushrooms in everything: soup, gravy, salads, and the family favorite, a simple panfry in garlic and butter served on homemade toasted bread. The key thing about eating wild mushrooms is to only pick what you know. Don't be all gung ho and just pick and eat anything—there's a chance you'll get poisoned and die. Try to learn from seasoned foragers in your area. There are even mushroom classes you can take, where an expert will guide you out into the field and show what is editable and what will make you sick.

The paddocks weren't the only source of free and easy bounty, as my brother and I found out early on. We discovered freshwater crayfish (yabbies) in the river that ran through our property and we'd catch them and boil them in a billy on a campfire for breakfast. Looking back, I realize now how fortunate we were to have access to this foraging wonderland. In my adolescence I wasn't even familiar with the term "forage," but now I embrace it. I relish the oncoming mushroom season, the excitement of discovering a new patch of stinging nettle, the joys of salty rock mussels at the beach, and the freshness of yabbies from the dams.

If you are a city dweller there's certain bounty to be found for the urban forager. The amount of fruit that falls to the ground from urban trees is frustrating, so I get out there and collect some of that free food that overhangs in laneways, alleys, and parks. Some local governments have planted herb and vegetable plots that people can harvest from on the way home from work. Parks are also up for a good spot of foraging, mostly nuts, fruit, and mushrooms. Explore your local surroundings and you might be surprised what you discover.

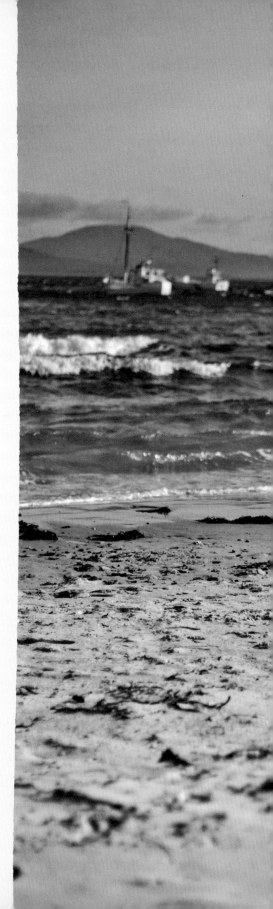

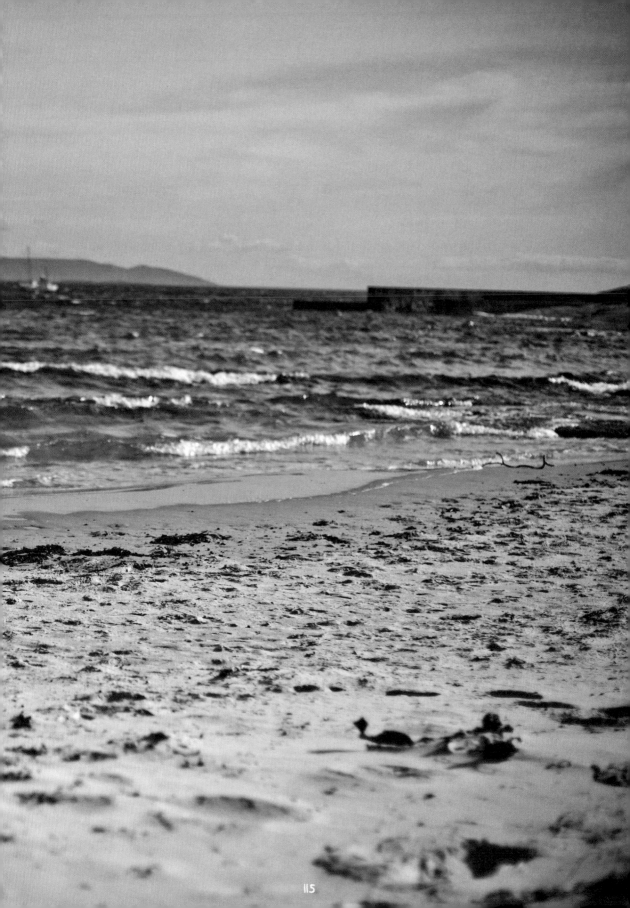

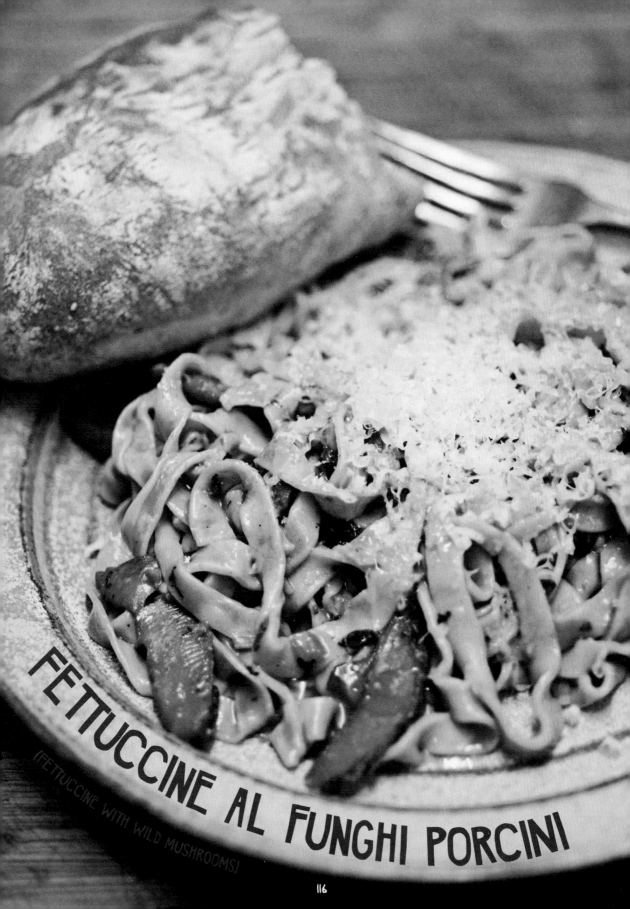

FETTUCCINE AL FUNGHI PORCINI

(FETTUCCINE WITH WILD MUSHROOMS)

AUTUMN BRINGS WITH IT MANY FORAGING OPPORTUNITIES, AND MUSHROOMING HAS TO BE ONE OF MY FAVORITES. FREE, TASTY, AND HEALTHY FOOD—WHAT MORE COULD YOU ASK FOR? IF YOU KNOW WHAT YOU'RE LOOKING FOR, YOU CAN ENJOY A RANGE OF WILD FLAVORS THAT YOU JUST DON'T GET FROM COMMERCIAL VARIETIES. BUT REMEMBER, WHEN PLANNING ON CONSUMING WILD MUSHROOMS, ONLY PICK WHAT YOU KNOW, LEAVE EVERYTHING ELSE ALONE. AND FOR A SUSTAINABLE HARVEST, ALWAYS CHOP THE MUSHROOM AT THE STIPE (STEM) TO ALLOW THE SPORES TO REGENERATE THE FOLLOWING SEASON.

TWO WILD MUSHROOM VARIETIES THAT ARE PROLIFIC IN OUR PINE FORESTS ARE EUROPEAN IMPORTS: THE SAFFRON MILK CAP AND SLIPPERY JACKS. THE SAFFRON MILK CAPS ARE A JOY TO COOK WITH.

THEIR NUTTY "JUST-PICKED-FROM-THE-FOREST-FLOOR" TASTE IS UNBEATABLE, AND THIS RECIPE IS SIMPLY ABOUT EMBRACING THOSE FLAVORS AND DOING LITTLE TO DISGUISE THEM. THE SLIPPERY JACKS ARE SLIPPERY, AND MANY PEOPLE MAY NOT LIKE THEM FOR THIS VERY REASON. BUT LIKE EELS, I THINK IF YOU CAN PUSH ASIDE THAT PERCEIVED ICKINESS YOU CAN ENJOY WHAT FLAVOR THEY HAVE TO OFFER. I JUST DON'T TELL PEOPLE I'VE PUT THEM IN THE PASTA UNTIL AFTER THEY'VE LICKED THEIR PLATE CLEAN AND ASKED FOR SECONDS.

IF YOU DON'T HAVE WILD MUSHROOMS IN YOUR REACH, THEN TRY A FARMER'S MARKET OR GET SOME AT A SMALL GROCER THAT HAS WILD VARIETIES. USE WHATEVER WILD VARIETIES ARE SAFE TO EAT IN YOUR LOCAL AREA.

WHAT YOU NEED:

6 x medium size wild mushrooms
1 lb (500 g) fettuccini pasta
   (freshly made if possible)
1 x small onion, diced
3 x cloves garlic, chopped
2 oz (50 g) butter
1/2 cup Parmesan cheese, grated
1/4 cup (50 g) pouring cream
   (optional)
1 cup white wine (Pinot Grigio if
   you have it)
3 tbsp extra virgin olive oil
1 handful fresh sage, chopped
1 handful fresh thyme, chopped
Salt
Pepper

HOW TO:

Chop and discard the mushroom stalks and then slice your mushroom the full length of the cap to make long slices.

Heat a large frying pan and heat your olive oil. Add your onion and garlic and sweat for five minutes on a medium to high heat, then add your fresh herbs.

Meanwhile, pop in your fresh pasta and cook al dente.

Now add your mushrooms and sauté for 8 minutes. At the end add your wine and cook out the alcohol for a further 5 minutes.

You will notice a sauce developing. Add your butter. Stir well and turn down the heat. You should now have a great smelling and looking mushroom sauce. Season with salt and pepper.

Just before your pasta is cooked, add the cream and the Parmesan to the mushroom sauce and stir in. It should now be nice and creamy.

You can add your pasta straight to your frying pan using tongs. Don't worry about pasta water getting into the pan; it will help make the sauce.

Stir the pasta and the sauce well.

Serve with a splash of olive oil, grated Parmesan, and a spot of crusty bread on the side. Oh, and don't forget a glass of wine!

FIELD-FORAGED RAGU

AFTER A GOOD MORNING SESSION PICKING MUSHROOMS IN THE FOREST, THIS IS A WELCOME MEAL THAT CAN BE COOKED QUITE EASILY OVER A CAMPFIRE, WHICH ADMITTEDLY MAKES IT TASTE AT LEAST 50% BETTER. THE INGREDIENTS ARE SIMPLE AND CAN EASILY BE BROUGHT ALONG INTO THE FIELD IN A CAMP BOX IN THE BACK OF YOUR CAR, ESPECIALLY BECAUSE IT'S AUTUMN AND THE TEMPERATURE WILL BE COOL ENOUGH TO TRANSPORT THE FRESH STUFF. IT'S REALLY NEAT TO BE ABLE TO COOK A MEAL WITH THE KEY INGREDIENT, THE WILD MUSHROOMS, ONLY BEING PICKED MOMENTS BEFORE.

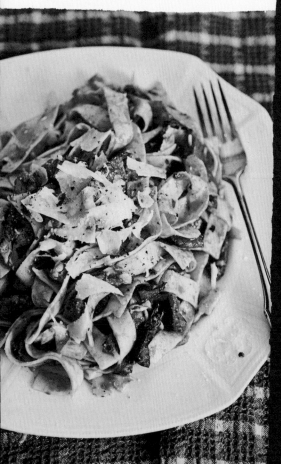

WHAT YOU NEED:

1 x chorizo sausage (or spicy salami...your choice)

Pasta (cooked of course, dried is far too crunchy)

3-4 x large saffron milk cap mushrooms (or any nutty wild mushrooms)

4 x cloves garlic

1 tbsp butter

Good quality Parmesan, pecorino, or Grana Padano cheese, grated

3 cups (700 ml) passata (see page 212)

1 glass red wine

1 handful fresh parsley, rough chopped

Extra virgin olive oil

Cracked sea salt

Cracked pepper

HOW TO:

Chop up your main ingredients—garlic, chorizo, mushrooms—and keep in separate bowls.

Heat a frying pan, pop in a good glug of olive oil, and the butter.

Add your chopped mushrooms and after a few minutes, when they look like they've had a bit of action, add your garlic and chorizo. The smell is unreal...yeah!

After a few more minutes, add your red wine, which will comprise the base for the sauce. Keep stirring it around with "delicate vigour." Let it cook out for a few more good minutes (don't panic these mushrooms are nothing like store bought mushrooms, they can take a bit of frying). It's at this stage that the mushrooms also take in all the flavor of the wine, sausage, and garlic.

Now add your passata, stir it well, and season the sauce with salt and pepper. Also add your parsley (set aside some for a garnish). Let the sauce simmer for a good ten minutes, keeping an eye on it so it's doesn't reduce too much. This is a good time to pop on your pasta.

Use tagliatelle, fettuccine, or even spaghetti—anything dry and easy to transport to the field. Drain the al dente pasta and return to the pot you cooked it in. Now add your sauce and mix it up well with the pasta.

Serve with a crack of pepper and salt, parsley, grated cheese, and a drizzle of olive oil.

NATURE IS A POWERFUL THING, WE JUST ACCEPT WHAT SHE DELIVERS.

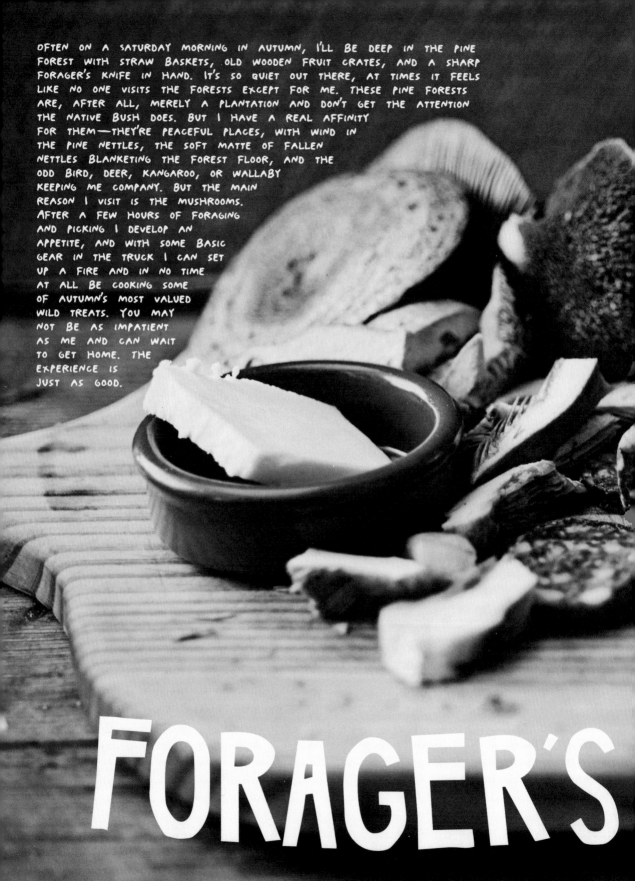

OFTEN ON A SATURDAY MORNING IN AUTUMN, I'LL BE DEEP IN THE PINE FOREST WITH STRAW BASKETS, OLD WOODEN FRUIT CRATES, AND A SHARP FORAGER'S KNIFE IN HAND. IT'S SO QUIET OUT THERE, AT TIMES IT FEELS LIKE NO ONE VISITS THE FORESTS EXCEPT FOR ME. THESE PINE FORESTS ARE, AFTER ALL, MERELY A PLANTATION AND DON'T GET THE ATTENTION THE NATIVE BUSH DOES. BUT I HAVE A REAL AFFINITY FOR THEM—THEY'RE PEACEFUL PLACES, WITH WIND IN THE PINE NETTLES, THE SOFT MATTE OF FALLEN NETTLES BLANKETING THE FOREST FLOOR, AND THE ODD BIRD, DEER, KANGAROO, OR WALLABY KEEPING ME COMPANY. BUT THE MAIN REASON I VISIT IS THE MUSHROOMS. AFTER A FEW HOURS OF FORAGING AND PICKING I DEVELOP AN APPETITE, AND WITH SOME BASIC GEAR IN THE TRUCK I CAN SET UP A FIRE AND IN NO TIME AT ALL BE COOKING SOME OF AUTUMN'S MOST VALUED WILD TREATS. YOU MAY NOT BE AS IMPATIENT AS ME AND CAN WAIT TO GET HOME. THE EXPERIENCE IS JUST AS GOOD.

FORAGER'S

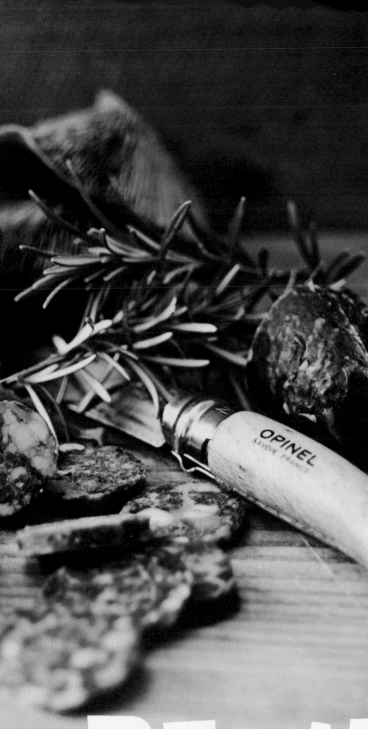

WHAT YOU NEED:

1/2 chorizo sausage
Pane di case
  (made the night before)
Mixed wild mushrooms
4 x cloves garlic
Splash of white wine
A few fresh sage leaves
A few sprigs of fresh thyme
Butter
Olive oil
Salt
Pepper

HOW TO:

Chop the mushrooms, chorizo, garlic, sage, and thyme.

Heat a frying pan. Add a knob of butter and a glug of oil.

When the butter is almost melted add all the mushrooms, and fry them for 5–10 minutes. When the mushrooms start to shrink and soften, add a splash of the wine, toss well, and cook for a few minutes more.

Season with cracked salt and pepper. Add the chorizo and the herbs, and simmer for a further 5 minutes to allow the flavors to be released.

Serve with some homemade bread and a warm thermos cuppa (that's tea to you Yanks).

REWARD

NETTLE PAPPARDELLE

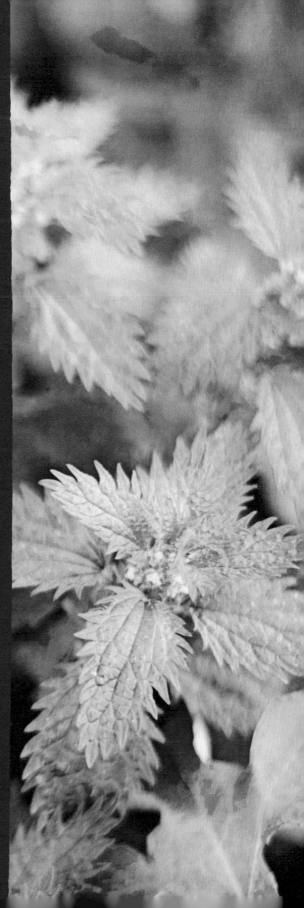

Sometime in the 1980s, my uncle John was just starting his career as a landscape gardener and he painfully discovered the toxic sting that the nettle will indiscriminately dish out to unsuspecting naked hands. I remember him telling us kids not to touch it; little did he know that years later I'd be eating it!

Stinging nettle has long been sought after for its health benefits and obviously, edibility. It is slightly spinach-like in flavor and will knock the socks off the most devoted carnivore. You will often find it in impoverished soil or under the shelter of large trees where the sheep take shelter. I carry a pair of rigger's gloves and garbage bags in the truck just in case I discover a patch, because it's gold and when it's available it's on the menu immediately.

WHAT YOU NEED:

large handfuls nettle
2/3 lb (300 g) pappardelle pasta
cup Parmesan cheese, grated
1/2 cup pine nuts, toasted
Olive oil
Salt
Pepper

HOW TO:

Panfry the pine nuts in a glug of olive oil for a few minutes until they turn slightly golden. Remove from pan when toasted.

Use tongs or gloves to place the nettle in a large pot. Boil it for a few minutes, and then pour out into a strainer. When the nettle has cooled down, squeeze out the excess liquid. (Don't worry about getting stung as the toxins are destroyed in the boiling process.)

In a food processor whiz up the nettle, cheese, and toasted pine nuts until you get a smooth consistency. Then slowly add some olive oil to turn the powder into more of a sauce.

Season to taste, and serve with al dente pappardelle.

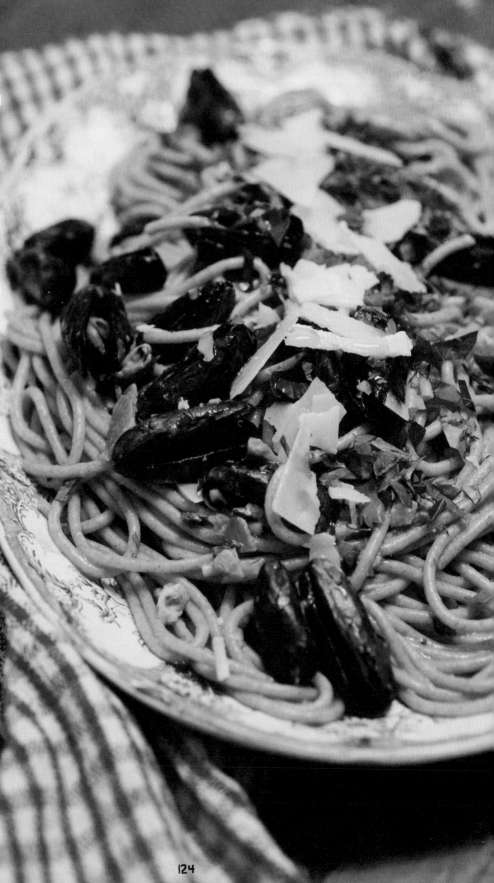

BEACHCOMBER'S PASTA

I'VE ALWAYS BEEN A FAN OF SEAFOOD MARINARA PASTA. FOR A LONG TIME IT WAS MY FIRST CHOICE AT ANY ITALIAN RESTAURANT. BUT OVER THE YEARS THE INGREDIENTS SEEMED TO BE GETTING MORE RUBBERY AND LESS FLAVORSOME, SO I DROPPED IT OFF THE MENU. I THINK THE PROBLEM LIES IN THE FRESHNESS (OR LACK THEREOF) OF CHEAP, FROZEN, IMPORTED SQUID AND PRAWNS. HOWEVER, THE LAST FEW SUMMERS I'VE BEEN CATCHING SAND CRABS AND SEARCHING THE BEACHES AT LOW TIDE FOR FRESH MUSSELS THAT CLING TO THE ROCKS, COLLECTING INGREDIENTS FOR THIS (NOW FAVORITE) SUMMER DISH.

SAND AND SHORE CRABS ARE A REAL DELICACY, AND THEY'RE NOT ABLE TO BE CAUGHT EVERYWHERE, BUT CHECK YOUR BEACHES FOR WHATEVER CRABS ARE AVAILABLE FOR CATCHING. LUCKILY, FOR ME, CATCHING CRABS IS RELATIVELY EASY. IN FACT THEY ARE CONSIDERED BY SOME FISHERMEN TO BE A PEST, AS THEY'RE OFTEN ON THE HOOK WHEN YOU'RE TRYING TO FISH FOR SOMETHING MORE, WELL, FISH-LIKE. THEIR MEAT IS AS SWEET AS LOBSTER (ALTHOUGH A BIT MORE TIME CONSUMING TO GET TO) AND THEY MAKE AN EXCELLENT STOCK.

WHAT YOU NEED:

3 x crabs (hand size)
1 lb (500 g) mussels, shell on
4 slices pancetta
Spaghetti/linguini
1 x lemon
5 x cloves garlic, chopped
3.5 oz (100 g) butter
1 cup white wine
1 x tbsp tomato paste
1 handful parsley
Olive oil
Salt
Pepper

HOW TO:

Boil some water in a pot, and cook the crabs until they change color, usually 5–8 minutes.

Remove and allow to cool. Remove the meat from the crabs. Set aside in a bowl.

In the same pot, return the empty crab shells, and 2 cups (a half a liter) of water and start making the crab stock. Leave the lid off the pot and simmer for 10 minutes. Remove and strain the liquid into a bowl, as this will be used to cook the mussels.

Boil salted water and start to cook the pasta.

In a frying pan, heat a glug of olive oil, and panfry the pancetta for a few minutes until crispy, then remove from the pan.

Check the pasta; when it's almost al dente, start the process of cooking the mussels.

In the pan, heat a little olive oil and add the garlic, allow to cook for a minute or two.

Now throw in the mussels and a ladle of the crab stock and also the white wine. Cover the pan with just enough of a gap for a little steam to escape.

After 5 minutes the mussels should be cooked. Add the butter to melt, and the tomato paste. Stir through.

Drain the pasta, and return it to the pot.

Add the cooked mussels, the crabmeat, crispy pancetta, parsley, and squeeze over the juice from the lemon.

Garnish with some parsley and a good grate of Parmesan and season to taste.

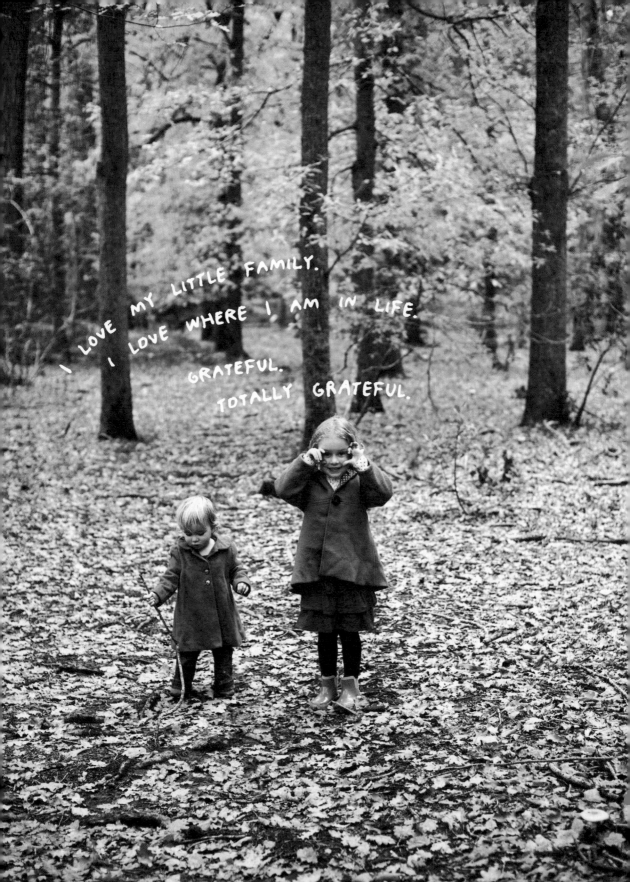

I LOVE MY LITTLE FAMILY.
I LOVE WHERE I AM IN LIFE.
GRATEFUL.
TOTALLY GRATEFUL.

SPUD + NETTLE SOUP

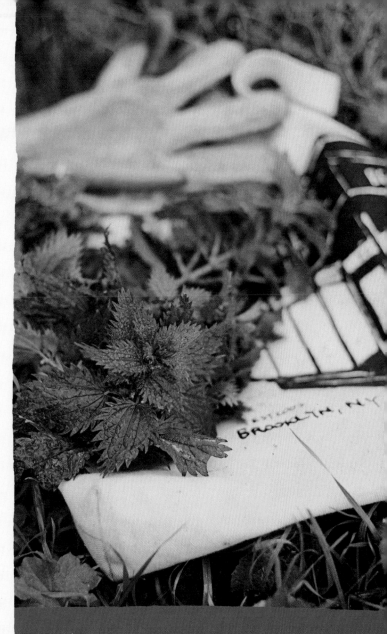

WHAT YOU NEED:

3 bunches fresh stinging nettle

3 x potatoes

1 x whole leek

5 x cloves garlic

1 quart (1 liter) chicken stock

Pouring cream

Knob of butter

1/2 tsp mace

Olive oil

Salt

Pepper

HOW TO:

Roughly chop the leek, garlic, and potato.

Heat a heavy based pot on medium; melt the butter along with a glug of olive oil.

Cook the leek and garlic for 10 minutes, until they're nice and soft.

Add the stock and a few cups of water. Increase the heat to high and bring the pot to a simmer.

Add the nettle and potato.

Add the mace and season.

Cook on a gentle simmer for 15 minutes, and then whiz with a stick blender.

If you're feeling evil, serve with a dollop of the naughty cream.

WHY WOULD YOU NOT WANT TO MAKE THE MOST OF A PLANT THAT GROWS WILDLY, IS FULL OF HEALTH BENEFITS, AND TASTES GREAT? JUST MAKE SURE YOU PICK WILD STINGING NETTLE WEARING GLOVES TO AVOID THE PAINFUL STING, AND YOU MUST BLANCH THEM FOR A FEW MINUTES BEFORE HANDLING THEM OR EATING THEM. THE FLAVOR IS UNMISTAKABLY SIMILAR TO SPINACH, SO CAN BE APPLIED TO MANY RECIPES IN PLACE OF SPINACH. IT SEEMS TO GROW ALL YEAR ROUND BUT IS AT ITS PEAK IN LATE WINTER AND THROUGH SPRING— A PERFECT TIME TO MAKE THIS STUNNING SOUP TO WARM THE TEMPERATURE-CHALLENGED COCKLES OF ANYONE'S HEART.

WALNUT FARFALLE

WALK DOWN AN URBAN BACKSTREET, INTO A PARK, THROUGH PADDOCKS, OR DOWN COUNTRY LANES AND THERE'S A HIGH PROBABILITY YOU ARE WALKING PAST FREE FOOD. I HAVE A MENTAL PICTURE OF WHERE ALL MY GOOD FORAGING SPOTS ARE; I'M A WALKING GPS UNIT. THE FORAGER'S CODE IS NEVER TELL ANYONE YOUR GOOD SPOTS. I'M HAPPY TO SHARE, AS LONG AS I KNOW WHERE YOU LIVE. IT'S AN I-CAN-TELL-YOU-BUT-THEN-I'D-HAVE-TO-KILL-YOU KIND OF THING.

OVER THE YEARS I'VE GOTTEN TO KNOW MY LOCAL HAUNTS FAIRLY WELL. IF YOU ASKED (AND AS I EXPLAINED, IT'S POLITE NOT TO) I COULD TELL YOU WHERE THERE IS A FIG TREE HANGING OVER A NEIGHBORHOOD FENCE; A PATCH OF NETTLE; AN INFESTATION OF SWEET BLACKBERRIES; A DARK FOREST VALLEY LADEN WITH MUSHROOMS; AND THE HIGHLY COVETED LOCATION OF MATURE WALNUT TREES. IT IS HIGHLY COVETED BECAUSE WALNUT TREES TAKE A VERY LONG TIME TO MATURE AND BECOME PROLIFIC PRODUCERS OF NUTS. IF KEEN FORAGERS KNOW ITS LOCATION, IT'S SURE TO GET A GOOD HAMMERING. EACH YEAR RAIN, HAIL, OR SNOW, I'LL DRAG THE KIDS OUT WITH BUCKETS AND COLLECT THE FALLEN NUTS AT ONE OF OUR SPOTS. LUCKILY FOR US THERE IS A PLAYGROUND NEARBY WHERE THE KIDS RETIRE AFTER FIVE MINUTES OF COLLECTING. I DON'T MIND. WE USUALLY MAKE A GAME OF WHO CAN COLLECT THE MOST IN THE LEAST AMOUNT OF TIME. BECAUSE THE NUTS HAVE BEEN OUT IN THE ELEMENTS, WE NORMALLY PLACE THEM IN THE ROOM WITH THE FIREPLACE, ON THE MANTLE, OR ON TRAYS ON THE FLOOR FOR AT LEAST A WEEK TO DRY THEM OUT.

IF I ACTUALLY HAD THE PATIENCE FOR BAKING I'D PROBABLY BE MAKING CAKES, SLICES, AND COOKIES. BUT THE WAY TO TREAT THESE BEAUTIFUL NUTS WITH THE UTMOST RESPECT IS BY MAKING A PESTO.

WHAT YOU NEED:

1 lb (500 g) farfalle

1 cup foraged walnuts (free just tastes better)

Large bunch fresh basil

1.5 cups Parmesan cheese, grated

1/4 cup olive oil

Salt

Pepper

HOW TO:

Warning: This meal may contain traces of nuts.

Crack the nuts open, remove the good bits, discard the shells.

Using a food processor mash the nuts to a fine consistency then set aside in a bowl.

Place fresh basil in the processor and whiz it up fine, then return the processed nuts and grated Parmesan.

Mix on a slow setting, while drizzling the olive oil into the processor.

Cook the farfalle al dente. When cooked and drained, return it to the pot it was cooked in and stir in the pesto. Mix well.

Serve with a good grate of Parmesan cheese, a dressing of olive oil, and cracked salt and pepper.

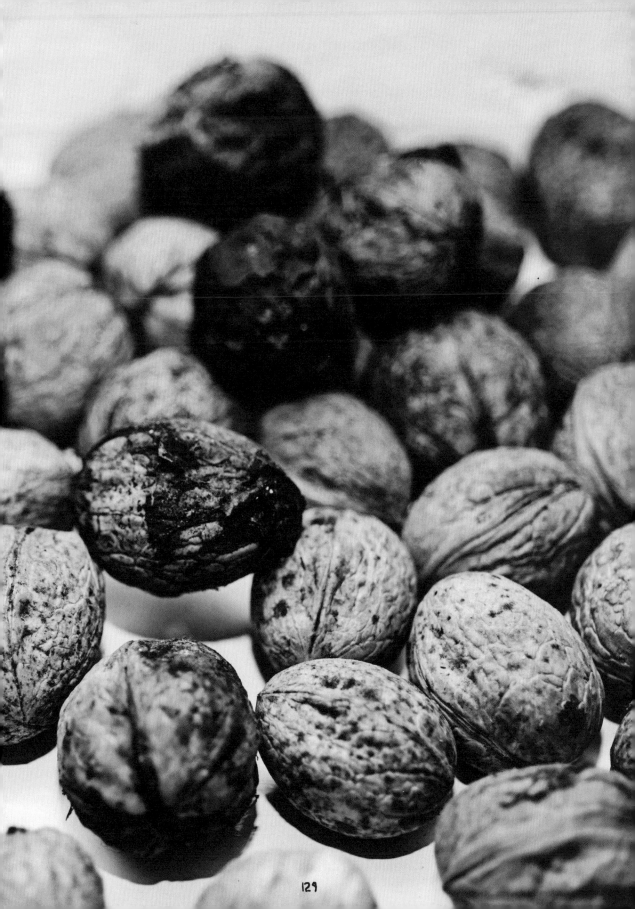

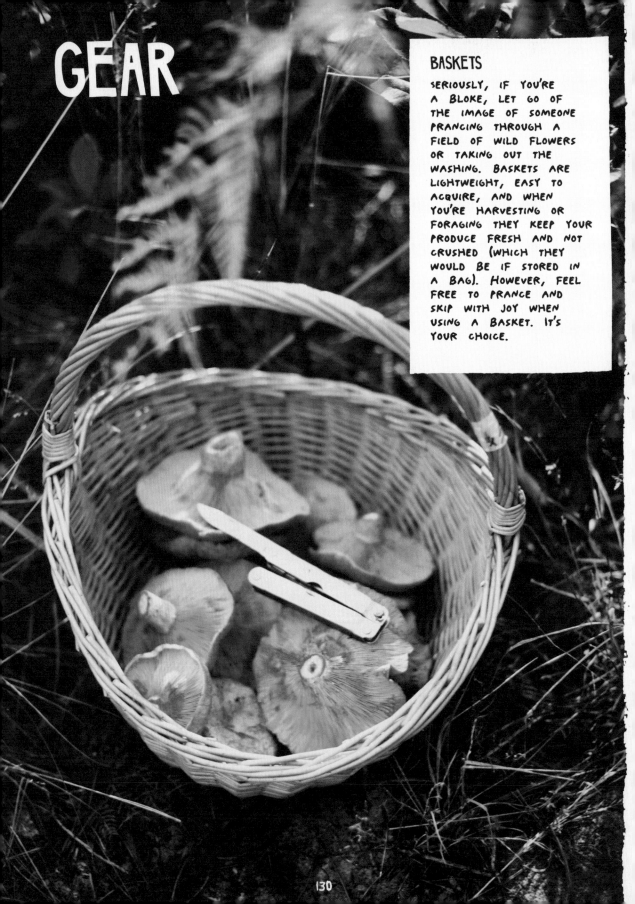

GEAR

BASKETS

SERIOUSLY, IF YOU'RE A BLOKE, LET GO OF THE IMAGE OF SOMEONE PRANCING THROUGH A FIELD OF WILD FLOWERS OR TAKING OUT THE WASHING. BASKETS ARE LIGHTWEIGHT, EASY TO ACQUIRE, AND WHEN YOU'RE HARVESTING OR FORAGING THEY KEEP YOUR PRODUCE FRESH AND NOT CRUSHED (WHICH THEY WOULD BE IF STORED IN A BAG). HOWEVER, FEEL FREE TO PRANCE AND SKIP WITH JOY WHEN USING A BASKET. IT'S YOUR CHOICE.

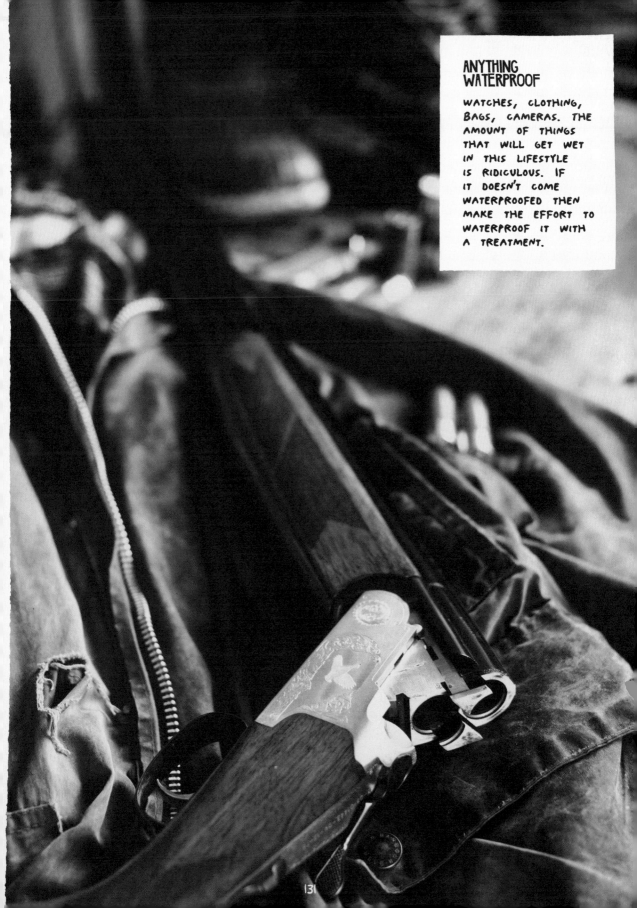

ANYTHING WATERPROOF

WATCHES, CLOTHING, BAGS, CAMERAS. THE AMOUNT OF THINGS THAT WILL GET WET IN THIS LIFESTYLE IS RIDICULOUS. IF IT DOESN'T COME WATERPROOFED THEN MAKE THE EFFORT TO WATERPROOF IT WITH A TREATMENT.

FROM THE FISHED

WILD:

For me, fishing was my initial foray into taking from the wild. Our little farm was blessed with river frontage, full of wild trout, eels, blackfish, and freshwater crayfish. For a teenage kid this was heaven. My older brother and I would often hunt for yabbies on weekends without the burden of school and chores; just the two of us out in the bush eating what would no doubt cost a small fortune at any decent restaurant. Every time I taste a Brie cheese made in that region, I can still taste the flavor of wild crayfish. There is something so unique about wild food!

The fishing I started out with was bare bones, worm on a hook with sinker, and fairly successful. The cooking was simple too. We baked trout and blackfish with butter and garlic in tinfoil, which led me to develop an appreciation for simple flavors that preserve the core ingredient.

Fishing is arguably an easier way to acquire a source of meat than hunting. You can walk into any sporting goods store, pick out a rod, and start fishing. Unfortunately, as a species, our love and hunger for fish has diminished wild populations in both sweet and salt water, so if you're going to fish be responsible. Only take what you need, leave the little ones in, and if you do catch a fish and you know it isn't going to survive then don't put it back in, that's a waste. I get so frustrated when I go fishing and see multiple dead trout washed up on a lake or river, obviously caught for "fun" and returned to the water after they're stressed, where they subsequently die. Imagine the stress fish go through being caught and taken out of their habitat. If you do fish for sport, then use a landing net, avoid touching the fish with dry hands, and get that fish back in the water as soon as possible.

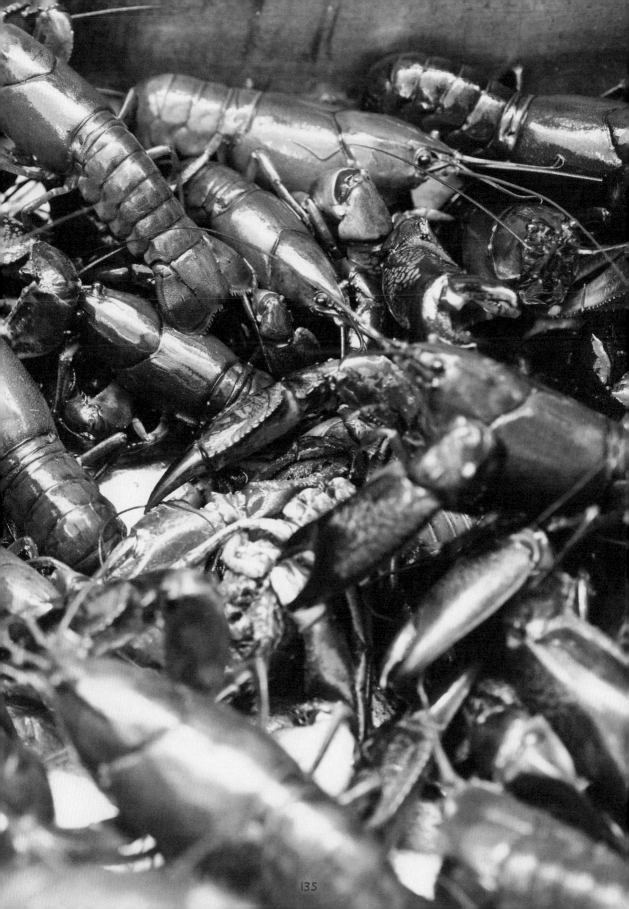

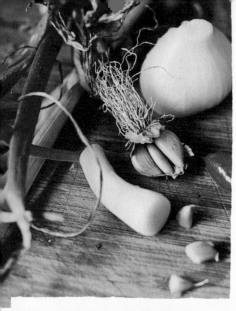
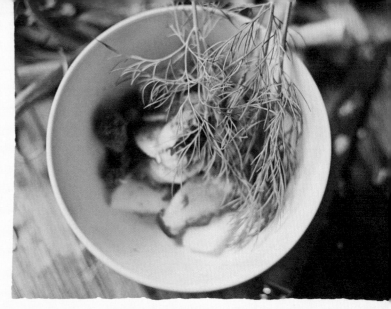
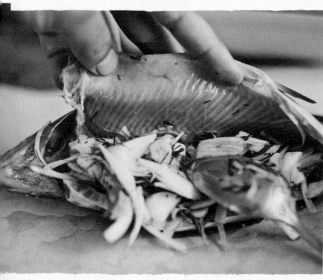
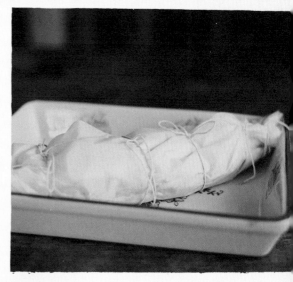
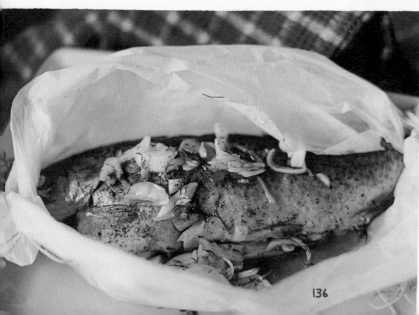
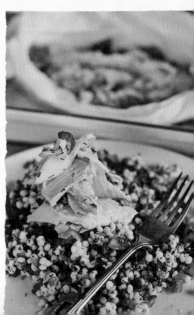

BAKED TROUT + TABOULEH

NEXT TO SMOKING TROUT, BAKING IS UP THERE AS ONE OF THE BEST WAYS TO TREAT THIS FISH. IF YOU'RE HANDY WITH A ROD OR HAVE ACCESS TO A TROUT FARM, ALWAYS TRY TO GET THE "PULL IT OUT OF THE WATER YOURSELF" VARIETY. THAT WAY YOU ENSURE FRESHNESS AND IT GETS YOU OUTSIDE AMONGST THE NATURE STUFF...IT'S WHERE YOU BELONG.

STEP ONE. CATCH FISH.

WHAT YOU NEED:

2 x fresh trout
1 x small onion
2 x spring onions (don't panic, you can grow them in
    summer...odd I know)
1 x fresh chili
4 x cloves garlic
1 x lemon, juice
1 handful fresh dill
1 x tbsp brown sugar

HOW TO:

Chop up the onion, spring onion, dill, chili, and garlic and place in a mixing bowl.

Mix in the sugar and lemon juice with all the chopped veg.

Place the trout in baking paper and stuff them with the mix. Place some mix on the outside of the fish.

Drizzle well with olive oil, and wrap up the baking paper to totally cover the fish. Tie up with baking string.

Bake for 15 minutes at 400 F (200 C).

Serve with tabouleh (see page 34) and drizzle the mix and any juice left in the baking paper over the fish.

GARLIC PRAWN RISOTTO

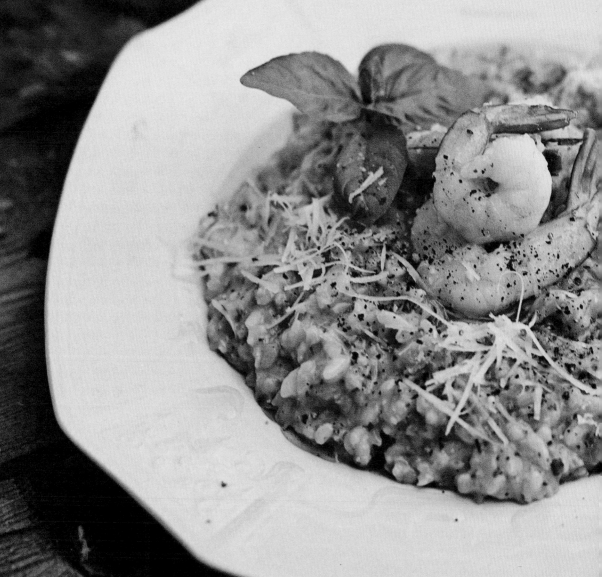

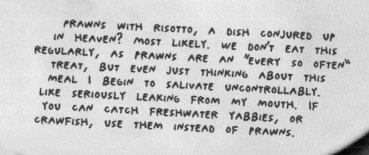

PRAWNS WITH RISOTTO, A DISH CONJURED UP IN HEAVEN? MOST LIKELY. WE DON'T EAT THIS REGULARLY, AS PRAWNS ARE AN "EVERY SO OFTEN" TREAT, BUT EVEN JUST THINKING ABOUT THIS MEAL I BEGIN TO SALIVATE UNCONTROLLABLY. LIKE SERIOUSLY LEAKING FROM MY MOUTH. IF YOU CAN CATCH FRESHWATER YABBIES, OR CRAWFISH, USE THEM INSTEAD OF PRAWNS.

WHAT YOU NEED:

2 lb (1/2 kg) raw, unpeeled prawns
Cooked risotto (see page 99)
6 x cloves garlic, diced
1/2 cup white wine
1/2 cup basil pesto (see page 208)

HOW TO:

Peel and clean the prawns. Slice along the back of the meat to remove the poo tube, and butterfly the meat.

When the risotto is resting, after you have placed the Parmesan and butter in and placed a lid on it...

Heat a frying pan with a splash of olive oil and add the garlic.

As the garlic begins to change color, add the prawns, for just a few minutes. They will change color to become less translucent and more opaque.

Pour them straight into the pot of risotto, and add the basil pesto. Stir well.

Serve with a dressing of olive oil, and garnish with fresh basil.

HOW + WHERE TO FISH

If you're thinking of fishing sweet water then there are three main approaches: live bait, spinning lures, and fly-fishing. Despite what the purists will tell you, all methods ARE successful in their own right. I started with live bait, then spinners, and now fly-fishing. This won't work for everyone but it's just how I've evolved behind the rod. I guess I've been fishing for so long I just wanted to "tackle" different methods (sorry I had to use it at some point). They all have their place, and live-bait fishing in the summer sitting next to a cold six-pack with good company is almost unbeatable. But then again, wading up an unexplored river in the high country, surrounded by stunning nature is also up there when it comes to life experiences and good times. The main idea is to get a few fish for the plate. How you do it is irrelevant as long as you do it responsibly.

If your state requires a fishing license, remember that this fee goes towards improving your fishing experience in the form of access gates, re-stocking, pest control, and population monitoring. Like hunting, always check with the local authorities before you pick up the rod.

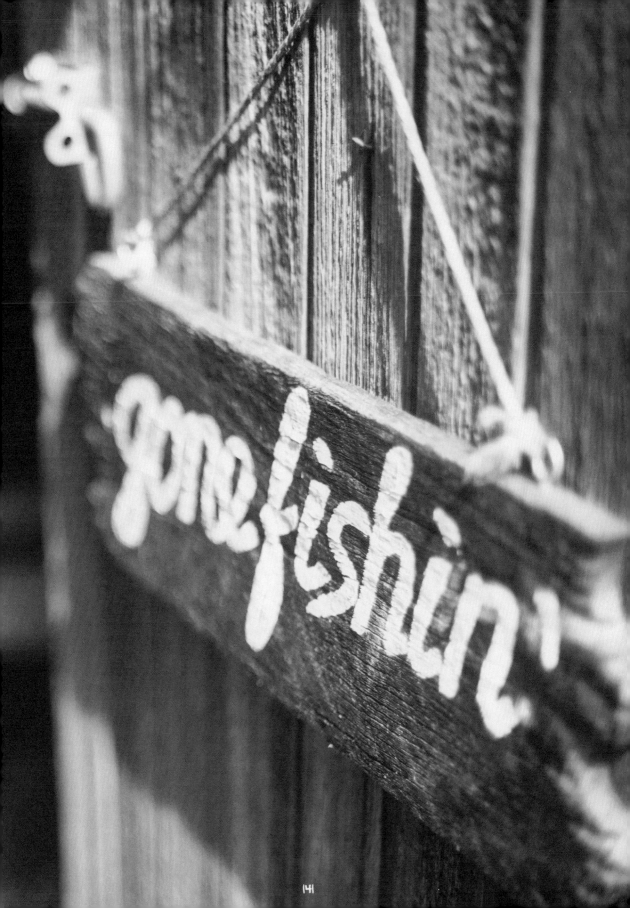

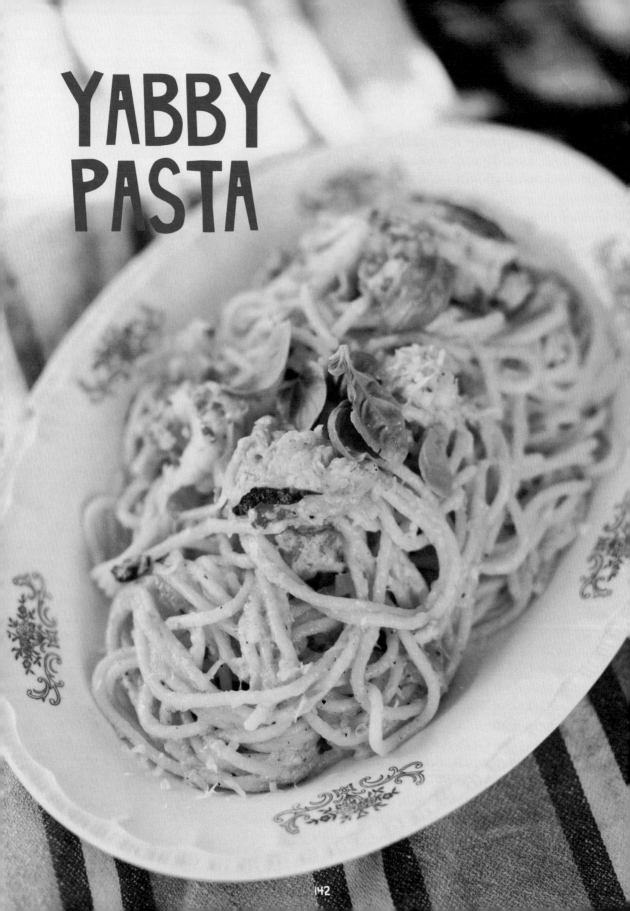

YABBY
PASTA

Catching "yabbies" is a childhood tradition I remember fondly. We'd head to someone's farm—I have no recollection whose place it was—on a mission: to trap the sweet-tasting, freshwater crustacean we call yabbies. In other parts of the world they might be called crayfish or crawfish, but for me and for our purposes they're still yabbies.

The normal approach was to boil large numbers at a time, crack open the shells, and devour the fresh meat like a gang of hungry hyenas. I'm not totally convinced that I've evolved much from that method, nor do I have any intentions to do so. Saying that I have, I cooked up some yabbies for some friends once, and they made a garlic butter sauce.

This dish is a tribute I guess, not the greatest sauce, just a tribute. As usual for me, it's a simple meal to make, and it's a treat for a summer's day when the weather's fine enough to eat outdoors with friends and family.

WHAT YOU NEED:

2 lb (1 kg) fresh yabbies (alive)

1/3 lb (150 g) smoked salmon

Orecchiette pasta

6 x whole garlic bulbs, diced

1 x lemon, juice

1 cup white wine

1 cup pecorino cheese, grated

2 tbsp Philly cheese

1 tbsp butter

1 small bunch fresh basil, roughly chopped

A few sprigs lemon thyme

1 tsp chili powder

Salt

Pepper

HOW TO:

Do the prep work; grate the pecorino, dice the garlic, chop the basil, and slice the salmon. Set aside separately.

Boil water in a large pot and cook the yabbies in small batches for a few minutes until they turn bright red. Set aside to cool.

Crack each yabby open and remove the meat from the tail and the claws. Rinse under water and place in a bowl.

In a large pot bring the water to boil, add a pinch of salt, add the pasta, and give it a good stir so the orecchiette doesn't stick.

While the pasta is cooking, heat a frying pan on medium. Add the butter and a glug of olive oil, then the diced garlic, lemon thyme, and white wine. Allow this to simmer on medium heat for 5 minutes.

Push the sauce from the frying pan through a steel, fine-mesh sieve into a bowl—this is flavor country! Return this flavorful sauce to the pan.

When the pasta is al dente, add the yabby meat, the salmon, and the fresh basil to the frying pan that has the sauce in it.

Now scoop out the pasta with a draining spoon and place it into the frying pan, mixing and turning over the sauce to coat the pasta. Add the Philly cheese and stir through until melted, then squeeze the lemon juice over the pasta. Continue to stir through so all the pasta is coated.

Serve with some fresh grated pecorino cheese, dress with olive oil and S&P, and garnish with some basil leaves.

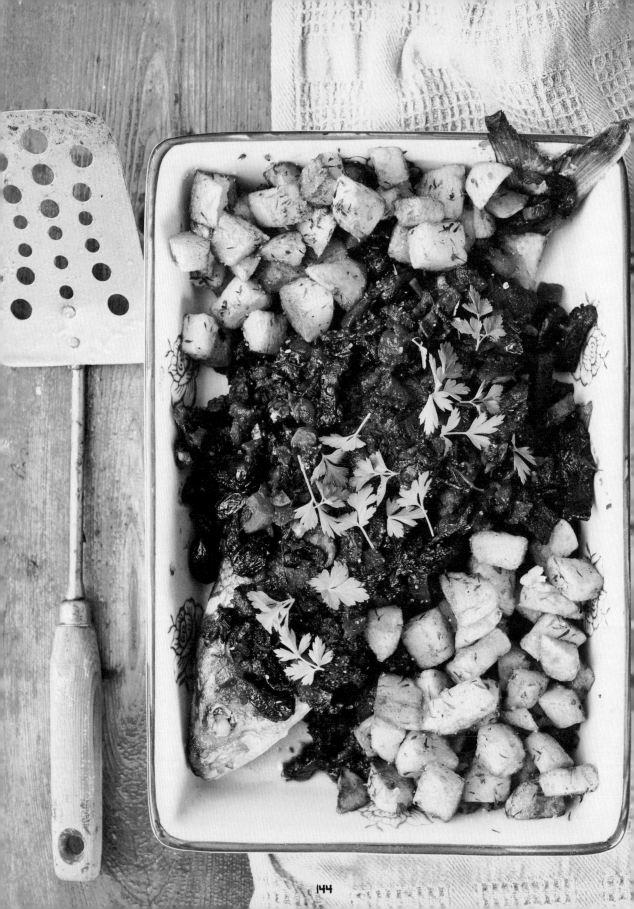

ARRABIATA FISH + CHIPS

ARRABIATA IS ONE OF MY REGULAR CHOICES WHEN I VISIT AN ITALIAN RESTAURANT FOR THE FIRST TIME. IF THEY CAN GET THAT RIGHT THEN YOU CAN GENERALLY JUDGE THE QUALITY OF THE PLACE. FOR ME, JOINING THIS SAUCE WITH FISH WAS INSPIRED BY THE ITALIAN WRITER ANGELO PELLEGRINI'S DESCRIPTION IN HIS BOOK *THE UNPREJUDICED PALATE*. HE WOULD DO SOMETHING SIMILAR WITH MOST FISH. THIS VERSION COULD BE APPLIED TO MANY FISH, BOTH SALT- AND SWEET-WATER, WITH PRETTY OUTSTANDING RESULTS...THAT IS, IF YOU'RE A FAN OF THE ARRABIATA IN THE FIRST PLACE! ADDING THE CHIPS ISN'T NECESSARY, BUT HEY, WE ONLY LIVE ONCE!

WHAT YOU NEED:

1 x whole fish (any whole fish around 1 pound)
5 slices hot salami, chopped
4 slices prosciutto, chopped
3 x large mushrooms, chopped
2 x onions, chopped
5 x cloves garlic, chopped
2 cups (500 ml) passata (see page 212)
1 cup red wine
Knob of butter
1 handful parsley, chopped
1 handful black olives
Tabasco sauce
Plain flour
Oilve oil
Salt
Pepper

Chips:
4 x potatoes, peeled and roughly cut into chunks
1 tbsp dried thyme
Cooking oil

HOW TO:

Preheat the oven to 350 F (180 C).

In a large pan, heat some olive oil and brown the salami and prosciutto on high heat until they get a little crisp, then turn the heat down to medium and add the onions. Cook them until softened.

Turn the heat up again, stir well.

Add the wine and deglaze the pan, scraping all the flavor goodness from the bottom. You should see a nice sauce forming.

After the wine had reduced almost completely, add the passata, mushrooms, garlic, olives, parsley, and a splash of Tabasco. Stir all ingredients through well and season.

Simmer on low for 20 minutes. If it reduces too much add a splash of water and stir through.

Wash the fish and pat dry, then dust both sides in flour.

Heat the butter and a glug of oil in a new pan on high heat and brown the fish on both sides. We don't want to fully cook the fish here, we just want to give the flavors a kick-start, so just a minute for each side.

In a baking dish, ladle out a spoonful of the sauce, place the fish on that and then spoon the remaining sauce over the fish.

Bake for 20 minutes.

Parboil the potato chunks for five minutes, then drain.

Heat about half a cup of cooking oil on high heat. When hot, place the potato in, and sprinkle over the dried thyme. Cook until golden brown.

Garnish the fish with fresh parsley and place the chips in the baking dish to serve.

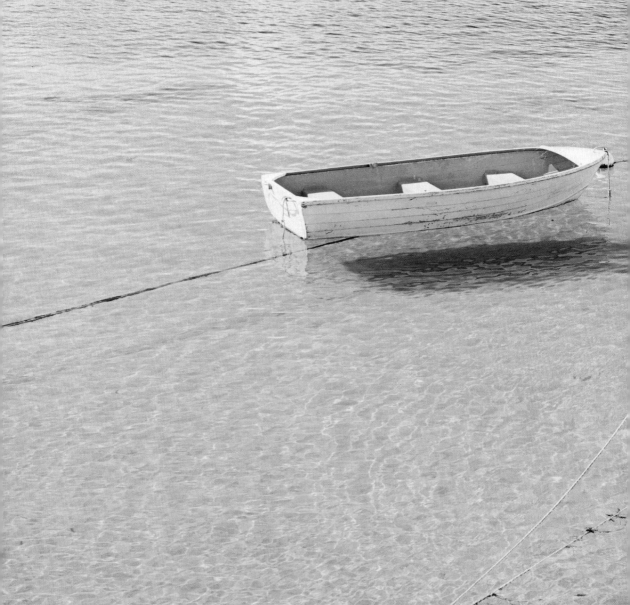

THIS FOOD REPRESENTS THE
IT REPRESENTS WHAT WE SHOULD HOLD ONTO TIGHTLY:
AND A DETERMINATION TO PROVIDE FOR
THESE ARE THINGS WE SHOULD

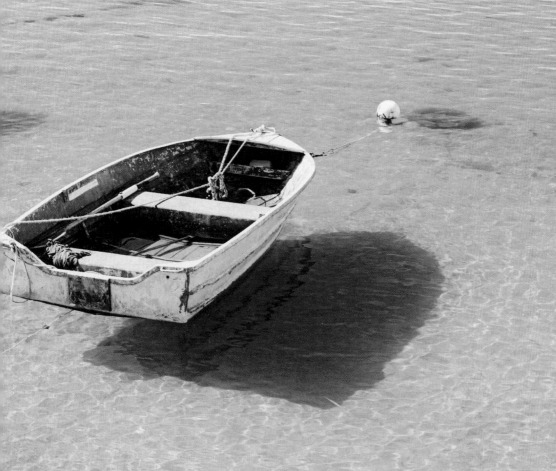

OLD WAYS.
TRADITION,
ONESELF.
TREASURE.

So the fishing gods where looking kindly upon you today: you've got your catch! The day cannot get any better than this. Oh wait, maybe a few gins could improve things, but that's beside the point. Some fish require removal of scales and all fish require the removal of guts.

First, run a fish scaler (which you can get all decent fishing shops) "against the grain," so to speak, while firmly holding the fish. Run tail to head until all scales have been removed, since you don't want to get a scale in the mouth when you've gone to all that effort to make a meal. I tend to use the trick of running cold water over the fish to wash off all the remaining scales. Without looking at the fish I'll run my hands over it. Using this approach of "seeing" with your hands you will find any remaining scales your eyes might have missed.

The guts need to be removed. Luckily, this is an easy job. Find the bum hole on the underside of the fish, usually at the end, near the tail fin. Push a sharp blade in the hole, pointing up towards the head and slice up to the neck. With the gut cavity open, grab all the guts and pull out in one rip, then rinse well under cold running water. You now have a perfect, wild fish ready for the pot, frying pan, or smoker.

PRE

PARING FISH

SUMMER'S CATCH PAPPARDELLE

THIS RECIPE CAN BE APPLIED TO MOST FISH, BUT IT'S PARTICULARLY EFFECTIVE FOR THOSE OF THE SALMONOID VARIETY. THAT BEING SAID, I HAVE MADE IT WITH A SMOKY BBQ-GRILLED BREAM AND THE RESULTS WERE EQUALLY PLEASING. I WONDER IF THAT IS MERELY BECAUSE I TOOK THE EFFORT TO CATCH THE FISH MYSELF?

WHAT YOU NEED:

Whole smoked fish, meat removed and de-boned,
   around 2 lb (approx 800 g–1 kg)
4 x slices of prosciutto chopped
1 lb (500 g) pappardelle pasta
1 x lime, juiced
1 x small, fresh chili, de-seeded and diced (optional)
4 x tbsp Philadelphia cooking cream cheese or
   pouring cream
1 x cup Parmesan cheese, grated
1 handful fresh dill or chervil, finely chopped
Garlic
Olive Oil
Salt
Pepper

HOW TO:

Pop the pasta in boiling, salted water.

Panfry the prosciutto and the garlic and set aside.

When the pasta is al dente, drain it and return it to the pot it was cooked in.

Add the all the ingredients, including the crunchy fried prosciutto and garlic, then mix well.

Serve with a dressing of olive oil and a sprinkle of fresh dill.

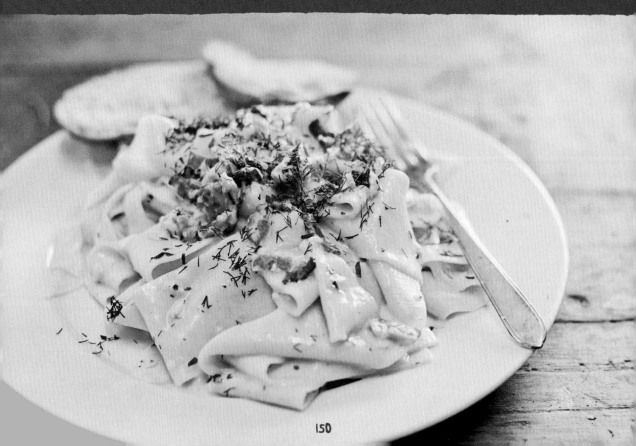

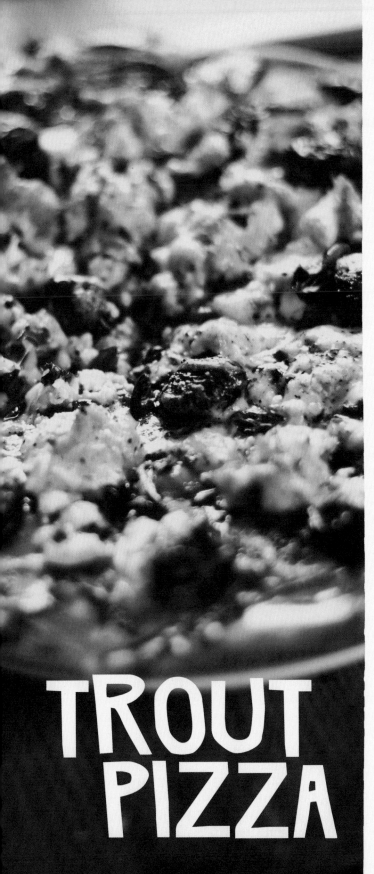

It might not seem like an obvious choice, but it works like a charm. The key for any decent pizza is having good quality ingredients, but not so many as to confuse the palate. Like most of my meals, I try to produce most of the ingredients, and this is no exception. Catch the trout, smoke the trout, pickle the olives, make the passata, grow the basil, grow the rocket... you get the picture.

Pizza Base:

28 oz (800 g) 00 flour (extra for dusting)
3 cups (700 ml) lukewarm water
1/2 oz (14 g) dry yeast
1 tsp caster sugar
Semolina flour

Toppings:

1 x whole smoked trout, meat removed and
   de-boned
1 handful rocket
Fresh basil
Olives
Roasted passata (see page 212)
Bocconcini
Marinated goats' cheese
Olive oil

How To:

Roll out the pizza base (instructions on page 230), and spread out the roasted tomato passata over the dough.

Add your toppings minus the rocket and basil. Drizzle with olive oil prior to cooking.

Cook pizza for 25 minutes at 350 F (180 C).

Serve with a generous garnish of rocket and basil and dress with olive oil.

TROUT PIZZA

EEL CAKE WITH WHITE BEANS

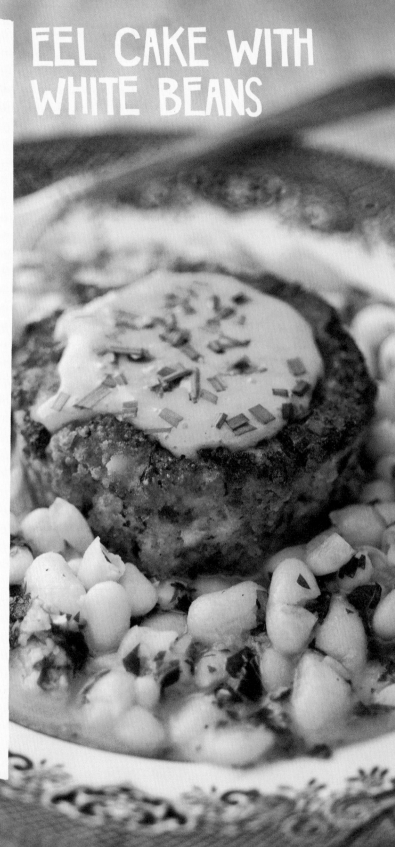

EEL, THE OTHER, OTHER WHITE MEAT.

FOR THIS RECIPE YOU COULD USE ANY FISH MEAT, BUT IF YOU'RE GAME, TRY THE EEL. FOR US IT'S THE EASIEST FISH TO CATCH ON A LINE. NO FLY ROD NEEDED, NO SPECIALIST SKILLS, JUST A GOOD OLD HAND LINE WITH A SQUIRMING WORM LEFT OVERNIGHT, SINCE EEL ARE NOCTURNAL HUNTERS. IF YOU HAVE A GOOD CATCH, AND A CRYOVAC, SMOKE ALL YOUR EELS. A GOOD CRYOVAC SEAL WILL KEEP THE SMOKED EEL FRESH FOR A FEW WEEKS IF REFRIGERATED.

INSTEAD OF SERVING THE EEL CAKE LIKE A FILLET OF FISH IN A BURGER BUN, OR WITH A BIG SALAD, A SERVE OF BUTTER WHITE BEANS THAT YOU GREW LAST SUMMER CAN BE THE PERFECT COMPLEMENT TO THE MEAL. GROWING CANNELLINI BEANS IS A MUST FOR US OVER SUMMER. WE LEAVE THE BEANS IN THE POD ON THE VINE, AND PICK THEM AT THE END OF SUMMER WHEN THE PODS HAVE DRIED AND THE BEANS ARE SUITABLY CURED FOR STORAGE. WE'LL REMOVE THE DRIED BEANS FROM THE CRACKLY DRIED PODS AND STORE THEM IN LARGE SEALED JARS FOR WINTER COOKING.

WHAT YOU NEED:

Eel Cakes (makes approx 6-8):

1/2–2/3 lb (200–300 g) smoked eel meat, diced
3 x eggs
5 x large potatoes
1 x onion, grated
1/4 cup Parmesan cheese, grated
1 tbsp fresh dill, finely chopped
1 tbsp fresh parsley, finely chopped breadcrumbs
Plain flour
Cooking oil (not olive oil)
Salt
Pepper

White Beans:

1 cup dried cannellini beans
1 x lemon
1/2 cup white wine
3.5 oz (100 g) butter
1 handful of parsley
Olive oil
Salt
Pepper

HOW TO:

THE EEL CAKES:

Boil the potatoes until they are soft enough to be pierced easily with a fork.

Strain, then mash the potatoes. Allow to cool.

Add the smoked eel meat to the potato mash, along with 1 egg yolk, parsley, dill, Parmesan, and grated onion.

Mix well with your hands, or if you're less adventurous use a large mixing spoon. However you do it, make sure you mix well to get an even spread of flavor throughout.

Whisk the remaining eggs in a bowl. Set aside.

Form the mash into small cakes and then lightly coat them on all sides with flour. Then coat the cake in the egg mix, and finally coat with the breadcrumbs as evenly as possible.

Panfry in hot oil until golden brown.

Serve with a dollop of aioli.

THE WHITE BEANS:

Soak in water overnight.

Boil them for an hour or until soft. Drain and rinse with hot, running water.

In a frying pan, melt half of the butter with a dash of olive oil.

Add the beans and parsley, and mix well. Then add the white wine and lemon juice and cook down for a few minutes while gently stirring. Cook some, but not all, of the liquid out.

Turn off the heat and add the last of the butter and more parsley and season with salt and pepper. Give it a flip and stir and serve when the butter has melted in to form a nice creamy base.

Serve with the cake, and drizzle the remaining juices over the beans.

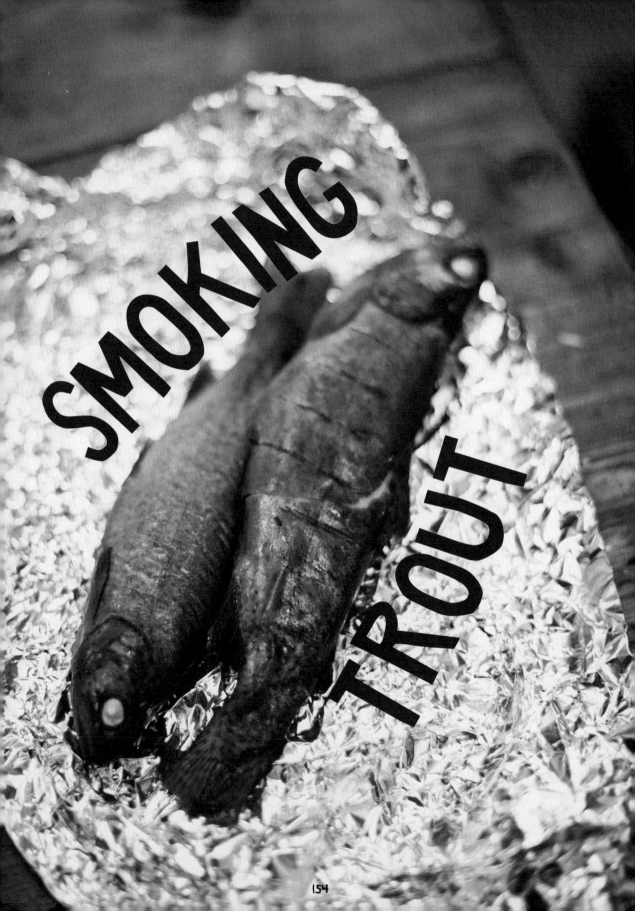

SMOKING TROUT

This is one of my favorite ways to cook. It's simple and the end result is one of life's little pleasures. Smoked trout/salmon/eel is loved by so many people, serving this up is sure to put a smile on any piscivore's face. The process hasn't changed much from ancient times. The principle is to use smoke to slowly cook the meat and infuse a smoky flavor throughout. Like most things in life, we tend to over-complicate. Ask someone how they smoke their fish and you'll get a totally different answer from every bloke you ask. And no, it's not blended with Port Royal, sitting between a few sheets of freshly licked Tally-Ho. There are two main ways to smoke fish: the slow smoke and the hot smoke. Both have outstanding results and both are relatively easy to accomplish. Slow smoking...well, the process is implied. It involves a few days in a smoking chamber exposed relatively cool smoke. The only problem with this process is the set up. Slow smoking equipment is a tad more sophisticated than what you need for hot smoking, thus hot smoking tends to be the more popular of the two options. This is my process for hot smoking. There are many others, but for me this simple method rules.

CURE THE FISH:

To give the fish a little something special, first I cure them. Again, there are two general approaches, one is to soak the fish in brine and the other is to apply a dry salt/sugar. Feel free to experiment.

THE DRY RUB:

Mix well 2:1 cooking salt to brown sugar.

Rub the mix all over the fish; on the skin and inside the cleaned cavity.

Place your fish in a sealed container and refrigerate overnight.

Pat dry with a paper towel prior to smoking.

THE BRINE BATH:

Place your fish in a pot or tub, and fill it with water until your fish is submerged.

Add a generous handful of cooking salt.

Soak for a few hours, even overnight

Pat dry prior to smoking.

WOOD CHIPS:

Here is where the smoke comes from. So that the wood chips don't burn too quickly, it's recommended that you soak them in water, anywhere from 30 minutes to overnight. The bigger the chips in size, the longer they'll need to be soaked. In regards to what chips to use, there are no hard and fast rules. You can use anything from Mesquite, Apple, Hickory, Maple, or even Stringybark.

THE KIT:

If you're new to the process, it's best to outlay the measly $50 and get a smoking kit from the fishing/outdoors store. These come in various shapes and sizes. The rectangle versions are a great option. They're easy enough to throw in the boot on the next fishing/camping trip and small enough to hide under the BBQ when not in use. They'll come with a small burner, in which you need to burn a flammable liquid, along the lines of methylated spirits (an odor-free version). Lay out the damp chips, then the fish rack, place the fish on the rack then light that baby up. All smoking units cook at different rates, and depending on wind conditions and the intensity of the flame the chips may burn hotter or cooler, so the cooking times will vary somewhat, but it should take somewhere between 10 and 15 minutes. When the fish skin is slightly blackened and peels easily from the sizzling meat you're looking at a smoked fish. If you like, you can place a knife into the meat to check for pinkness. If you think it requires more cooking pop the lid on and give it another 10 minutes. With time, you'll get to know your smoking unit. They all have their own personalities. Crack open a nice ale, and soon enough you'll be tasting that beautiful smoked fished and telling tall tales about the one or two that got away.

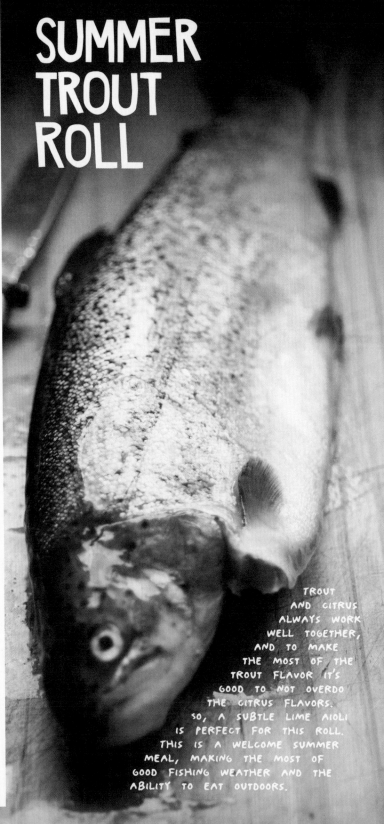

WHAT YOU NEED:

4 x trout fillets
Soft burger buns
Cucumber
Rocket
Fresh dill
Soft provolone cheese, sliced

Aioli Sauce:
3 x egg yolks
2 x cloves garlic, diced
2/3 cup light olive oil
1 tsp lime juice
1.5 tsp Dijon mustard
Salt
Pepper

HOW TO:

Put the eggs yolks, mustard, and lime juice in a mixing bowl and use an electric beater to mix. Slowly add the olive oil a little at a time until it begins to thicken. Don't rush when adding the olive oil: less is more.

Still mixing on a slow setting, add the diced garlic.

Season with salt and pepper.

Refrigerate the aioli.

Panfry/BBQ the trout fillets (use a bit of olive oil).

Spread the aioli on the base of the bun. Lay on the cooked trout, cheese, a slice or two of cucumber, and finally, a few rocket leaves.

Season with salt and pepper.

SUMMER TROUT ROLL

TROUT AND CITRUS ALWAYS WORK WELL TOGETHER, AND TO MAKE THE MOST OF THE TROUT FLAVOR IT'S GOOD TO NOT OVERDO THE CITRUS FLAVORS. SO, A SUBTLE LIME AIOLI IS PERFECT FOR THIS ROLL. THIS IS A WELCOME SUMMER MEAL, MAKING THE MOST OF GOOD FISHING WEATHER AND THE ABILITY TO EAT OUTDOORS.

WHAT YOU NEED:

1 lb (400-500 g) lox/salmon
1 lb (500 g) casarecce pasta
1 bunch fresh asparagus
1 tbsp dill, finely chopped
1 x lemon
1 cup pecorino, grated
3 oz (100 ml) pouring cream
Garlic
Olive oil
Salt
Pepper

HOW TO:

Smoke the fish as per your smoker's instructions.

When the fish is smoked and cooked completely, remove the meat and discard the skin and bones. Set aside in a bowl.

Cook the pasta in salted boiling water.

Halfway though cooking the pasta, blanch the asparagus in boiling water for 5 minutes. Drain and set aside.

When the pasta is al dente, drain and return to the pot it was cooked in.

Add the grated cheese, cream, chopped dill, and the smoked fish.

Grate half the lemon rind into the pasta and squeeze the juice out of the lemon. Mix well.

Serve with a portion of the blanched asparagus on top for each serve.

Dress with olive oil and some thin slices of pecorino and garnish with some chopped dill.

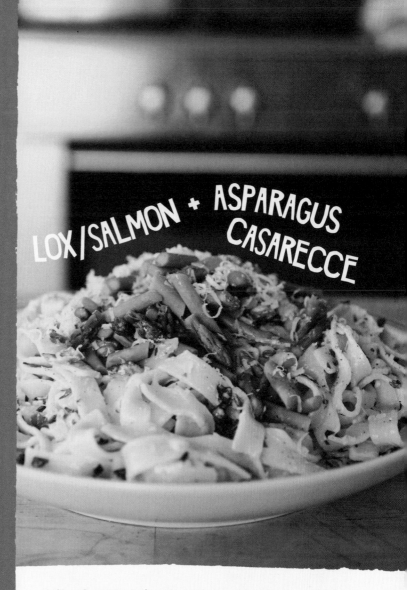

LOX/SALMON + ASPARAGUS CASARECCE

ONE OF THE JOYS IN LIFE IS DEVOURING SMOKED FISH, ESPECIALLY THOSE OF THE SALMONOID VARIETY. IF YOU'RE HANDY WITH THE ROD AND HAVE THE CHANCE TO GET OUT ON THE WATER IN SEASON, THEN TREAT YOURSELF WITH THIS LITTLE BEAUTY.

THERE ARE PLENTY OF SMOKERS OUT THERE... A BAD HABIT, YOU KNOW. YOU CAN GET A READYMADE HOT SMOKER STARTING AT AROUND $30, OR YOU CAN MAKE ONE YOURSELF (GOOGLE WILL TEACH YOU). IN ANY CASE THEY ALL WORK DIFFERENTLY, BUT ALL PRODUCE SOMETHING SMOKED AND DELICIOUS. GET TO KNOW YOUR SMOKER'S ABILITIES AND LIMITATIONS. IF YOU DON'T FISH YOURSELF THEN BUY YOUR FISH AS LOCALLY AS POSSIBLY AND FROM SOMEPLACE REPUTABLE.

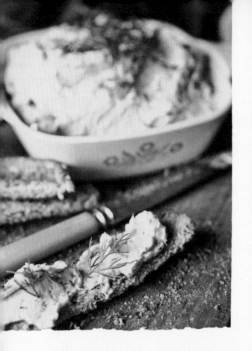

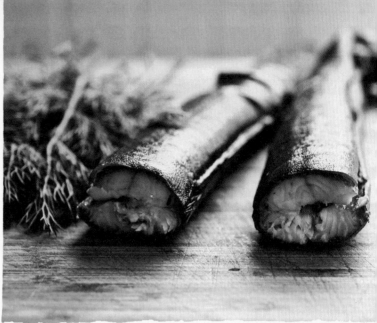

PEOPLE HAVE THIS STRANGE AVERSION TO EELS—SOMETHING ABOUT THEM BEING SLIMY AND SNAKE-LIKE, OH, AND APPARENTLY ELECTRIC. IT'S A VERY POOR JUDGMENT, FOR SUCH HIGH VALUE MEAT. IN MANY PARTS OF THE WORLD IT'S CONSIDERED A RARE DELICACY. IN FACT, MORE EEL IS EXPORTED TO ASIAN COUNTRIES THAN IS CONSUMED HERE.

YOU CAN TREAT EEL THE SAME WAYS YOU TREAT MOST FISH: BAKED, FRIED, PICKLED, AND USED IN SOUPS. BUT MY FAVORITE WAY TO ENJOY IT IS SMOKED. ITS TASTE IS NOT TOO DISSIMILAR TO OTHER SMOKED FISH, AND I'VE OFTEN WONDERED IF PEOPLE CAN TELL THE DIFFERENCE BETWEEN SMOKED EEL AND SMOKED TROUT. SO, I'VE BEEN MAKING THIS DISH TELLING EVERYONE THAT IT IS TROUT, AND EVEN THE FOODIES HAVEN'T PICKED UP ON IT YET. DO I HAVE HORNS GROWING OUT OF MY HEAD RIGHT NOW? YES I DEFINITELY DO. I'M A DEVIL OF AN EEL LOVER.

SNEAKY EEL DIP

WHAT YOU NEED:

1/2 eel

1 x lemon

7 oz (200 g) Philadelphia cream cheese

1/2 cup pecorino, grated

1 small bunch fresh dill

Olive oil

Salt

Pepper

HOW TO:

Smoke the eel. I slice it down the center from head to tail and butterfly it so that it gets an even smoking.

Allow the eel to cool, then remove the meat from the bone. Be sure to remove any rogue bones from the bowl of eel meat.

Finely chop the dill and set aside.

Using a stick blender, whiz up the eel meat in a bowl until paste-like.

Add the cream cheese to the bowl, the grated pecorino, along with a squeeze of lemon, and finally the chopped dill. Stir well and season with salt and pepper.

Transfer into small bowls and refrigerate for a few hours prior to serving.

And remember, the key is a good poker face. "Sure it's trout.... Eel? Are you crazy?"

FOOD IS NOT SUPPOSED TO BE STRESSFUL.
IT'S SUPPOSED TO BE GOOD FOR THE SOUL.
THUS I'D NEVER MAKE IT AS A CHEF.

I COOK, LET'S LEAVE IT AT THAT.

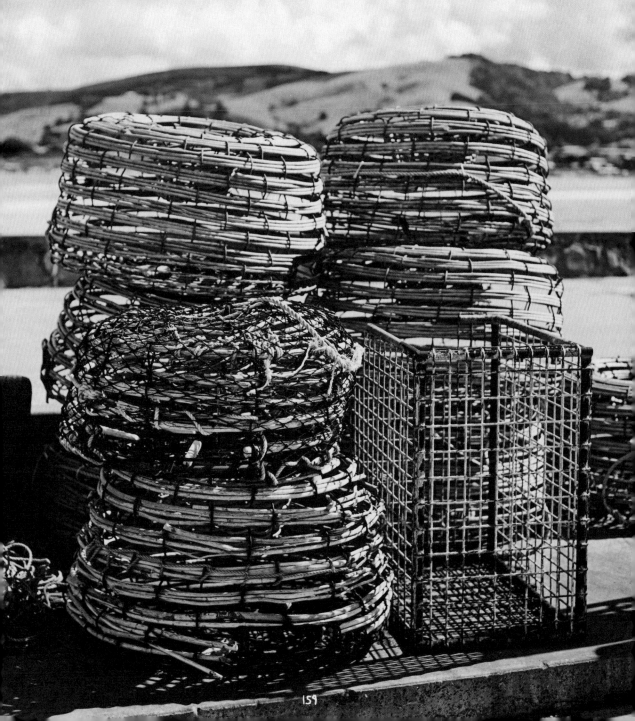

COAL-BAKED BREAM

AFTER A FULL DAY OF FISHING, THERE'S NO BETTER WAY TO REWARD YOURSELF THAN BY SITTING AROUND A CAMPFIRE WITH EXCELLENT COMPANY AND A COLD FROTHY IN HAND. IT COULD BE OUT IN THE BUSH, IN A CABIN, OR ON THE SAND. THERE'S A PRIMEVAL SENSE OF CAPABILITY, OF BEING ABLE TO HUNT YOUR FOOD AND COOK IT SIMPLY. BEFORE YOU'VE HAD TOO MANY COLDIES AND START TO SING SEAS SHANTIES AND TELL GHOST STORIES, TAKE THE TIME TO COOK SOME OF YOUR CATCH AND GET INTIMATE WITH THE FLAVOR OF THE WATERS. WHETHER YOU'VE BEEN WORKING THE ESTUARY OR THE SALTY STUFF, THE FISH SPECIES YOU CATCH WILL HAVE A UNIQUE TASTE THAT IS OFTEN DISGUISED BY BATTER OR HEAVY CONDIMENTS. A SIMPLE COOK/STEAM IN SOME WINE WILL KEEP IT SIMPLE, ALLOWING YOU TO APPRECIATE THE BASIC FLAVOR OF YOUR FISHY FOE.

AT THE HEIGHT OF SUMMER I LIKE TO FISH THE ESTUARY WATERS AND TARGET THE SWEET TASTING BREAM, WHICH COOK UP BEAUTIFULLY WITH THIS SIMPLE TREATMENT. BUT YOU CAN COOK ANY FISH THIS WAY AS LONG AS YOU HAVE ENOUGH ALUMINUM FOIL.

WHAT YOU NEED:

Patience and skill to catch the damn fish (a fishing rod also helps)

1 x whole bream (or other fish: snapper, mullet, flathead, etc.)

Lemon

Knob of butter

White wine

1 small bunch of dill

Cracked salt

Cracked pepper

Aluminum foil

HOW TO:

Light a fire. The temperature of the coals is important, so have the fire going for a while and set aside a bed of coals just on the outskirts of the main fire.

Gut and scale the fish then rinse under cold water. Place it on a sheet of foil.

Chop up the dill and slice the lemon.

Spread some butter on the outside of both sides of the fish and pop some in the cavity.

Place dill and lemon in the cavity, and if you have some remaining, place on the outside of the fish.

Drizzle a few tablespoons of white wine on and around the fish, this will help it steam.

Season with salt and pepper.

Fold in all the sides of the foil to create a sealed package. Place it on the bed of coals while placing some coals on top of the fish envelope.

Because there is no temperature gauge on a campfire, it's impossible to say how long to let it cook for. It's normally around 10 minutes.

Serve with jacket potatoes also wrapped in foil and placed on the coals 20 minutes prior to cooking the fish.

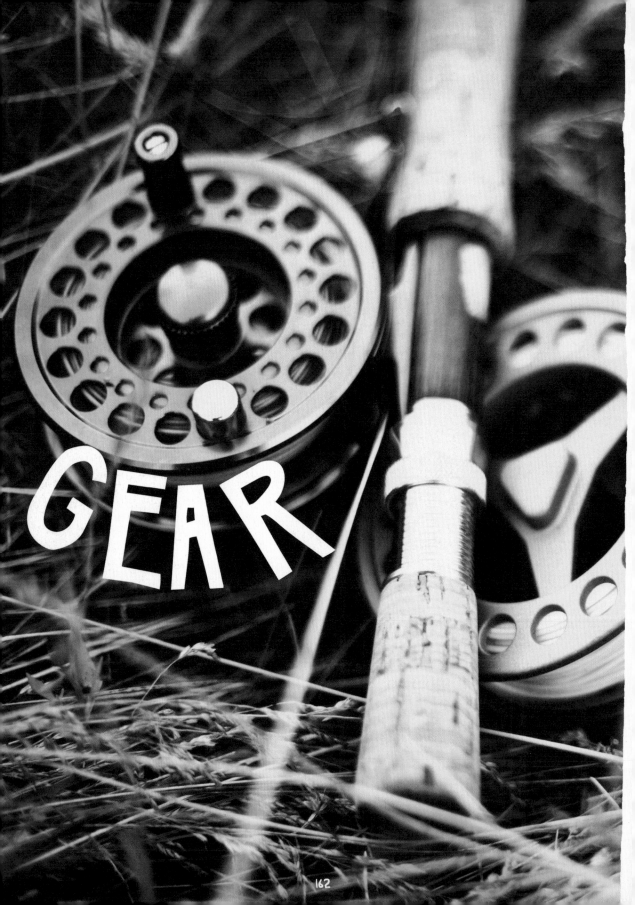

GEAR

FLY PATTERNS

THERE IS MUCH TO DISCUSS ON THIS TOPIC SO MUCH
THAT ENTIRE BOOKS ARE WRITTEN ON THE SUBJECT.
FISHERMEN/WOMEN DEVOTE THEIR ENTIRE LIVES TO
MAKING THE PERFECT FLY OR FINDING THE FLY BEST
SUITED FOR THEIR FAVORITE RIVER. I USE A FEW
DIFFERENT TYPES AND MY FLY BOXES ARE FULL, BUT
THAT'S NOT BECAUSE I'M TRYING TO OUTDO OTHER
FISHERMEN. IN FACT I HAVE MANY LESS THAN THE
PROS OUT THERE. BUT THE DRIVING IDEA IS THAT
WHEN YOU HIT THE WATER YOU WANT TO HAVE
OPTIONS. PICKING THE RIGHT FLY FOR A PARTICULAR
STRETCH OF WATER IS AN ART FORM IN ITSELF.
YOU HAVE TO ENGAGE IN A BIT OF DETECTIVE WORK.
LOOK AT THE WATER, WATCH TO SEE TROUT FEEDING,
ARE THEY FEEDING ABOVE THE WATER LINE ON
FLOATING FOOD LANES OR ARE THEY STAYING DOWN
AND FEEDING ON MACRO-INVERTEBRATES AND NYMPHS?
TROUT TEND TO FEED ON WHAT EVER IS THE MOST
ABUNDANT AND WHAT EVER WILL COST THEM THE
LEAST IN ENERGY EXPENDITURE. THE SEASONS ALSO
DICTATE WHAT FLY YOU'LL TEND TO GET SUCCESS
WITH. IN WINTER THE BUGS ARE MOSTLY IN THE
LARVAE STAGE AND STILL DEVELOPING UNDER WATER,
SO USING A NYMPH PATTERN MIGHT WORK WELL. IN
SUMMER WHEN THOSE INSECTS HAVE HATCHED THEY
MAY BREED AND RETURN TO THE WATER TO DIE.
OR THEY MIGHT BE ABUNDANT AS THEY EMERGE
SOMETIME IN SPRING AND ARE STRONG ENOUGH TO
BREAK THE VISCOUS BORDER. IT'S COMPLEX. BEST TO
GO OUT WITH A GUIDE OR READ A LOT OF BOOKS. I
STARTED WITH THE LATER, THEN GOT HELP. ONE WEEK
WITH AN EXPERIENCED FLY-FISHERMAN AND I LEARNED
ROUGHLY THE EQUIVALENT OF A YEAR'S WORTH OF
BOOK-TAUGHT TECHNIQUE. BY THE END OF THE WEEK I
WAS CATCHING TROUT WITH MY EYES CLOSED... WELL,
NOT LITERALLY. THAT COULD HAVE BEEN DANGEROUS.

FLY FISHING BAG

I LOVE MY FISHING
BAG. I COULD USE A
VEST WITH ALL THE
MODERN POCKETS, AND
UV PROTECTION, AND
BREATHABILITY, ETC.,
BUT I JUST ADORE
MY CLASSIC BRADY
BAG. AN ENGLISH GEM
THAT HAS SERVED
THIS FISHERMEN FOR
A DECADE, THE BAG
I USE HAS A LINED
INTERNAL POUCH TO PUT
THE FISH AND HAS
ENOUGH ROOM FOR A
WATERPROOF CAMERA,
SOME DRINKING WATER,
LUNCH, AND A PHONE
FOR EMERGENCY, OH
AND OF COURSE THE
POCKETS ARE FULL OF
FLY BOXES, LEADERS,
AND LINES. BRADY
MAKES VERY GOOD
QUALITY BAGS, WHICH
I THINK ARE JUST
BRILLIANT. I HAVE
A SOFT SPOT FOR
TRADITIONALLY MADE
ITEMS OF SUPERB
QUALITY. YOU MIGHT
PAY MORE BUT IT WILL
LAST YOU A LIFETIME.

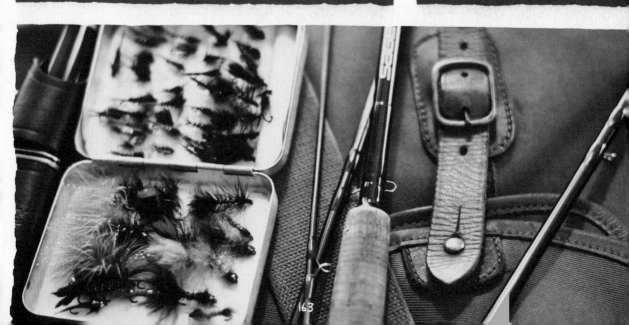

ROD—FRESH WATER

I USE A SAGE, 9-FOOT, SIZE #6 FLY ROD AND IT SUITS MY FLY-FISHING NEEDS. IF I WERE GOING TO FISH SMALLER STREAMS, THEN I'D LOOK AT A SIZE 4, AND IF I LIVED ON THE COAST OR FISHED BIG WATER I'D GO A SIZE LARGER THAN #6. BUT THIS SIZE WORKS WELL IN MY RIVER AND FOR MOST RIVERS THAT I TRAVEL TO. THERE ARE SO MANY FLY ROD BRANDS TO CHOOSE FROM, AND THEY ALL DO A JOB RELATIVE TO THE PRICE. WHATEVER YOU DO, JUST DON'T FALL INTO THE TRAP OF BECOMING A FLY-FISHING BRAND-OHOLIC. REMEMBER THAT FLY RODS USED TO BE MADE OUT OF VERY SIMPLE MATERIALS AND STILL CAUGHT FISH, SO SPENDING THOUSANDS ON GEAR WON'T MAKE YOU CATCH ANY MORE FISH.

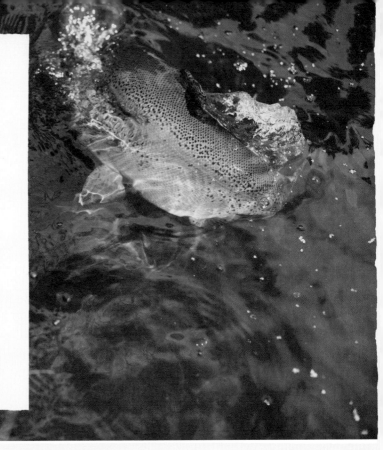

ROD—SALT WATER

I TEND TO FISH THE COAST OFF TIDAL ROCKS, SANDY BEACHES, AND OFTEN OFF PIERS AND JETTIES. FOR THE SURF AND ROCKS I USE A MASSIVE SURF ROD, THE ROD ITSELF IS BASIC BUT I DID BUY A DECENT REEL. SALT WATER IS A BITCH ON CHEAP REELS. A DECENT REEL MAKES ALL THE DIFFERENCE IN REGARDS TO LONGEVITY. TO HELP WITH MAINTENANCE, I WASH THE REEL UNDER FRESH WATER AFTER A SESSION. FOR FISHING OFF A JETTY I TEND TO USE A TRIGGER TIP LIGHT ROD AND REEL COMBO. I STEER CLEAR OF BAIT-CASTERS; THEY'RE A BITCH TO USE UNLESS YOU KNOW HOW TO CAST THEM WITHOUT GETTING A BIRD'S NEST OF TANGLE. STICK TO THE BASIC AND TRADITIONAL CASTING REEL.

WADERS

I HAVE FOUR SETS OF WADERS. I KNOW IT SEEMS EXCESSIVE, BUT THERE IS A REASON. TWO PAIRS ARE THICK RUBBER OVERALLS WITH RUBBER BOOTS ALL IN ONE. PERFECT FOR STANDING IN LAKES SHOOTING DUCKS, BUT NEARLY USELESS WADING OVER SLIPPERY RIVER ROCKS FLY FISHING, ESPECIALLY IN SUMMER WHEN THE SUN HITS THE RUBBER AND YOU BECOME A WALKING HOTHOUSE. THE OTHER TWO PAIRS ARE MADE BY ORVIS AND HAVE NEOPRENE BOOTIES THAT ALLOW YOU TO SLIP ON A PAIR OF FISHING BOOTS. THESE WADERS COME IN HIP- AND FULL-LENGTH OVERALLS (FOR THE DEEPER WATER). BOTH HAVE THEIR PLACE AND BENEFITS. THE PAIR I TEND TO USE THE MOST IS THE FULL-LENGTH, ORVIS CHEST WADERS. THEY DO IT ALL. THEY'RE BREATHABLE AND COMFORTABLE, AND THE ORVIS BOOTS I USE HAVE REMOVABLE STUDS THAT COME IN HANDY WHEN FISHING OVER SLIPPERY ROCKS.

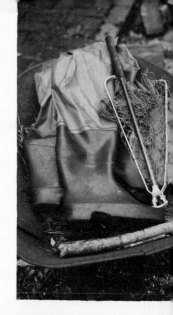

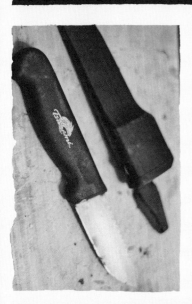

SCALING KNIFE

WHENEVER YOU GO FISHING BRING ALONG A FEW KNIVES. DEPENDING ON WHAT YOUR TARGET FISH IS YOU MAY NEED TO SCALE IT. YOU WILL DEFINITELY NEED TO GUT IT AND THIS IS BEST DONE IN THE WATER YOU'RE FISHING IN. THE ENTRAILS CAN FEED ANIMAL LIFE BACK IN THE WATER AND YOU WON'T GET INTO TROUBLE FROM YOUR LIFE PARTNER WHEN GUTTING A FISH IN THE KITCHEN SINK. I USE A FISHING KNIFE THAT HAS A SCALER EDGE ON THE BACKSIDE. IT'S AN EASY JOB TO SCALE A FISH. JUST GO AGAINST THE GRAIN MAKING SURE YOU GET ALL THE SCALES OFF. I TEND TO CLOSE MY EYES AND USE MY HANDS, FEELING ALL OVER THE FISH WHILE WASHING OFF THE REMAINING SCALES UNTIL THE FISH IS CLEAN. THERE IS NOTHING WORSE THAN A MOUTHFUL OF SCALES WHEN EATING FISH.

FILLETING KNIFE

DEPENDING ON YOUR TARGET FISH YOU MAY NEED A FILLETING KNIFE IF YOU DON'T PLAN ON COOKING THE FISH WHOLE. WHEN I FISH FOR SNAPPER, FLATHEAD, AND BREAM I TAKE THE FILLETING KNIFE OR AT LEAST HAVE IT BACK AT THE CABIN FOR WHEN IT'S TIME TO PREPARE THE FISH. THE DIFFERENCE BETWEEN A FILLETING KNIFE AND A KITCHEN KNIFE IS FLEXIBILITY, AND THEY'RE NORMALLY RAZOR SHARP IN ORDER TO MAKE CLEAN CUTS IN THE FLESH. SPEND A BIT ON THIS TOOL AND YOU'LL THANK YOURSELF IN THE FUTURE. HACKING A FISH TO PIECES WITH A BLUNT KNIFE IS NOT ONLY FRUSTRATING BUT WRECKS ALL THE HARD WORK YOU PUT INTO GOING FISHING IN THE FIRST PLACE.

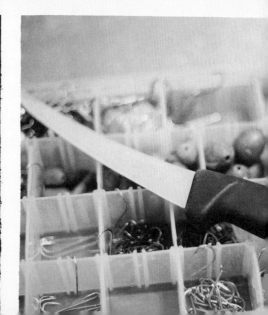

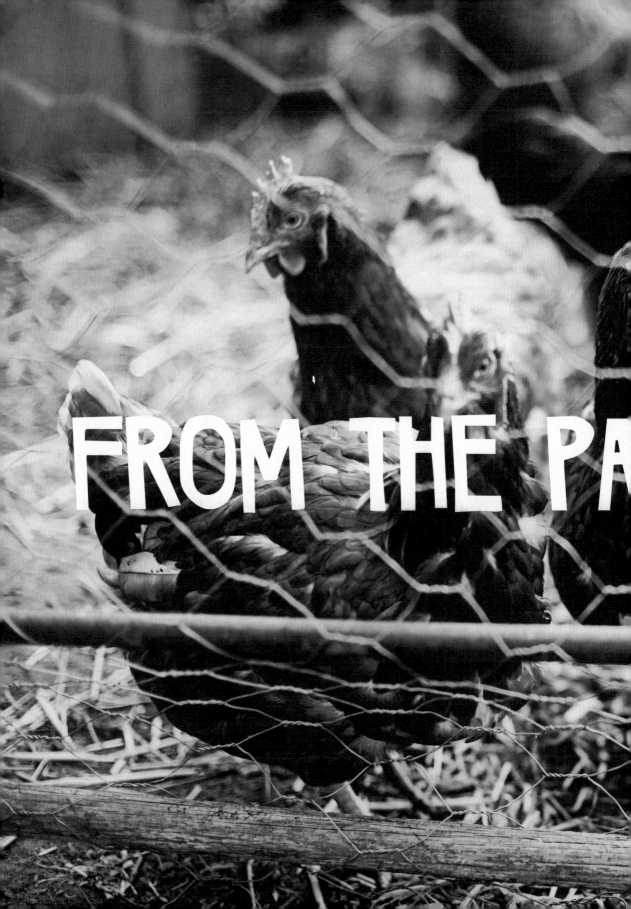

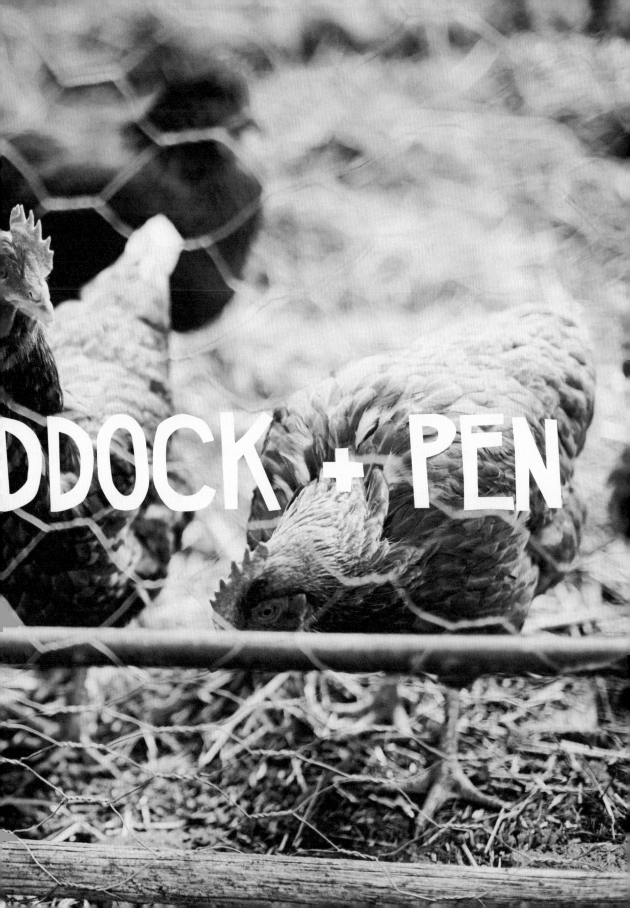

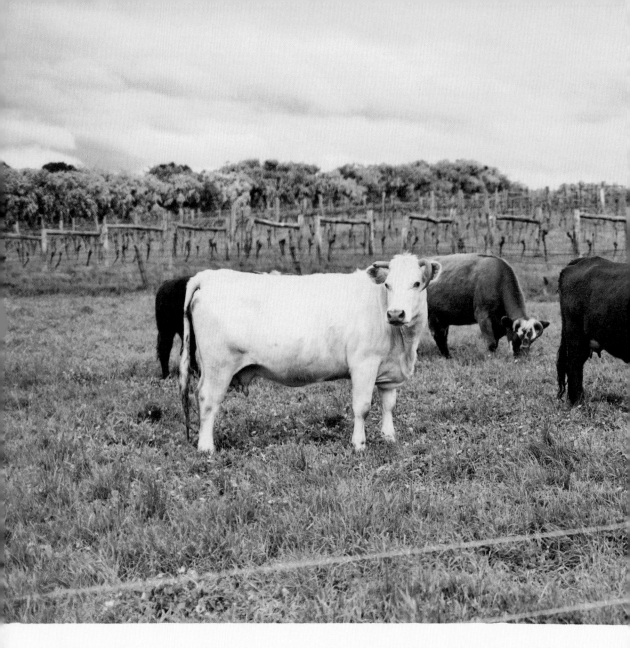

The production of red meat requires a lot of cleared land, and our insatiable demand for the stuff has had a very detrimental impact on our environment. All over the world land is still being cleared to make way for grazing, especially in developing countries where cheaper meat is the preferred choice of multinational food chains. Cattle and sheep grazing on such a huge scale is devastating to the natural population of so many species through habitat loss, reduced biodiversity, and soil degradation. And it's all a result of big companies trying to make a buck. But there is hope. If we reduced the amount and regularity of our red meat consumption, we'd surely help to at least slow these negative impacts.

In our home we view red meat as a special treat. We'll have maybe five lamb roasts a year, less for beef. Instead, when we eat farmed meat, we rely on local, free-range pork, chicken, venison, kangaroo, and duck—all of which have much less impact on the natural world. I'm not saying we don't enjoy red meat. It's bloody divine! It's just that we've shifted our habits. And when we do

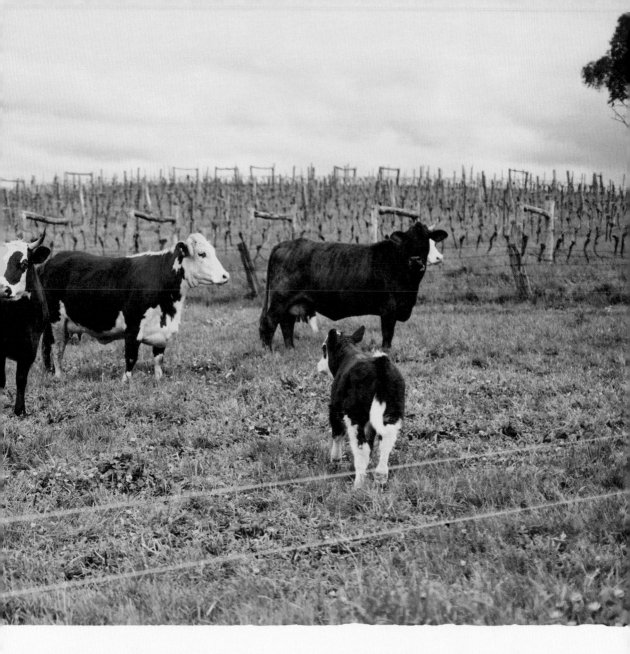

eat the red stuff, it's in a way that celebrates flavor of a beast that's been treated well.

In regards to the other farmed meats, there is such a good range to choose from, and in many cases you can even meet the people that raised it. There is a farmer at our local market who's started to raise free-range pigs. He is so passionate about his new farming endeavor that he regularly shows me photos of his setup when I visit him at the market (he also makes the best chorizo!) There are people out there doing great things when it comes to meat

production, and it's up to us consumers to support them. If you can't hunt or raise you're own meat, I suggest you eat less of it and source it wisely. You'll be helping the environment, local business, and you'll be rewarded with better quality, too!

Here are just a handful of recipes. Since you probably cook with these meats often there's no need for me to teach you something you already know. These are simply some examples of what we do with our meat when we get the call from a farmer friend or after a visit to the market.

INVESTING IN A CAST IRON CAMP POT WAS A WISE MOVE. FOR ONLY $50 I HAVE A COOKING POT THAT WILL LAST MY LIFETIME AND WILL BE SOMETHING I CAN PASS DOWN, JUST LIKE THE CAST IRON FRYING PAN THAT MY GRANDFATHER BOUGHT FOR MY MUM AND THAT I NOW USE EVERY WEEK. CAST IRON COOKWARE WORKS SO WELL BECAUSE IT RETAINS THE HEAT EVENLY AND CAN WITHSTAND A GOOD OLD BEATING. COOKING IN A CAMP POT (SOMETIMES REFERRED TO AS A DUTCH OVEN) IS AN OLD TRADITION, AND THERE IS A GOOD REASON FOR THIS—ITS SIMPLICITY. THERE ARE TWO WAYS TO COOK USING ONE OF THESE POTS: WITH DIRECT FLAME OR IN A BED OF COALS. I PREFER THE LATTER. SLOW COOKING CHEAPER CUTS OF MEAT LIKE A LAMB SHOULDER RESULTS IN SOFT, TENDER MEAT WORTHY OF ANY HIGH PRICED RESTAURANT. THE KEY IS THE FLAVOR YOU CHOOSE TO ACCOMPANY YOUR MEAT. WITH LAMB, THE BEST-MATCHED ROASTING FLAVORS ARE ROSEMARY, THYME, GARLIC, AND WINE.

THE KEY TO A GOOD, SLOW COOK ON A CAMPFIRE IS CONSISTENT HEAT FROM THE COALS; THIS IS ACHIEVED BY BUILDING A WELL-STOCKED CAMPFIRE, THUS CREATING A GOOD SUPPLY OF HOT COALS. GET THE FIRE ROARING FOR A GOOD HALF HOUR, AND THEN PLACE THE POT INTO A SMALL PIT NEXT TO THE MAIN FIRE. THE PIT BECOMES YOUR LITTLE OVEN, AND BEING NEXT TO THE FIRE ITSELF, IT'S EASY TO SHOVEL FRESH COALS ONTO THE POT WHILE IT IS COOKING.

THIS METHOD REALLY EMBRACES YOUR INNER PRIMITIVE MAN/WOMEN. BUT ONCE YOU'VE TASTED MEAT COOKED THIS WAY YOU WILL LONG FOR COLD WINTER AFTERNOONS IN THE BUSH, COOKING CHEAP CUTS OF MEAT IN YOUR POT.

CAMP-COOKED LAMB SHOULDER

HOW TO:

With a sharp knife make stab insertions all over the shoulder, and insert garlic cloves (from one garlic bulb) and sprigs of rosemary.

Drizzle a good portion of olive oil (around 2 tbsp) in the pot making sure the base is well covered so the roast will not stick.

Rub olive oil onto the roast and sprinkle to cover with dried thyme, cracked black pepper, and sea salt. Place the roast in the pot with the wine and water and the skinned cloves of your second garlic bulb.

Your cooking pit should be wider than your pot by at least 6 inches to allow for placement of fresh coals during the cooking process.

Place a thick bed of coals at the base of the pit then place the pot on top.

Shovel more hot coals around the base of the pot and some on top of the lid. Keep fuelling the main fire with more wood to ensure a steady flow of hot coals for the pot.

After about 40 minutes, carefully remove the lid and check the liquid level. There should be liquid in the pot, about halfway up the meat, maybe less. If required, add more water. The key is that it's not bone-dry, as the meat will spoil and be as tough as a dead dingo's donga. While the lid is off, add all of your vegetables. Return the lid and shovel fresh coals around the pot.

This is not a fine art and every fire is different, so keep an eye on the pot, removing the lid as you go to peek inside and check the progress. You don't need to cover the entire pot with hot coals, as this will make the pot too hot. The best way to cook the shoulder is slow and at a consistent temperature. The slower the better...more time to drink a glass or two of the Pinot brought to the fire!

Normally the roast will be cooked in around 2 hours, depending on the heat of the coals. To test if the meat is cooked place a skewer deep in the thick part of the meat, if red juice pours out then continue cooking, if it's relatively clear then the meat needs to be removed from the pot, wrapped in aluminum foil and rested for 10 minutes. Also remove the vegetables and cover.

Leave the remaining juices in the pot and return it to the fire with the lid off. Add the cornflour and stir and reduce to make gravy. Pour this over the meat and veggies.

Serve with a nice glass of Pinot Noir—that is, if there's any remaining!

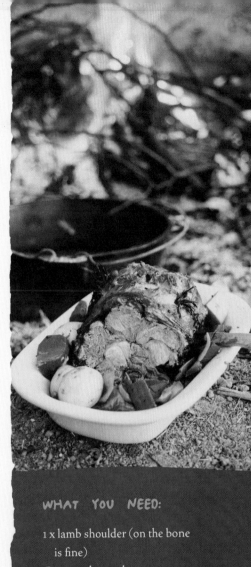

WHAT YOU NEED:

1 x lamb shoulder (on the bone is fine)
Carrots, chopped
Potatoes, chopped
Pumpkin, chopped
3 cups red wine
3 cups water
2 x whole garlic bulbs
1 large bunch rosemary sprigs
1 x tbsp dried thyme
Cornflour
Olive oil
Salt
Pepper

DARK + STORMY SHANKS

WHAT YOU NEED:

4 x lamb shanks
   ("Frenched" if you want
   to be fancy)
5 x medium mushrooms
   (wild if you can forage them)
2 x carrots
2 x parsnips
2 x sticks celery
1 x onion
5 x cloves garlic
24 oz (700 ml) stout
1/2 cup red wine
2 sprigs fresh rosemary
1/2 cup plain flour
2 tbsp cornflour
Water
Olive oil
Salt
Pepper

HOW TO:

Preheat the oven to 300 F (150 C).

Roughly chop all the vegetables and mushrooms and finely chop the rosemary. Set aside with the mushrooms separated out from the rest.

Cover the shanks in the regular flour and brown for a few minutes in a frying pan with some olive oil and half the chopped rosemary. When done, set aside to cool.

In the same pan (now empty) fry the mushrooms and deglaze with the red wine. Cook the mushrooms until they reduce in size (around 5–8 minutes) then remove.

In a large oven dish, heat some olive oil and sauté the vegetable mix for 10 minutes on a medium heat. Stir well.

Place the shanks on top of the veg, along with the cooked mushrooms. Then add the beer and the other half of the rosemary. If necessary top off with water to cover the meat. Season.

Bring to a simmer.

Place the pot in the oven, covered. Cook for an hour, then remove from the oven and check the fluid levels. If the liquid is low add hot water to cover the meat. Spoon mix the ingredients and return to the oven for another hour.

When the meat is falling off the bone, remove the shanks into a serving dish and cover with tin foil.

Place the pot on the stove and pop in the cornflour. Reduce to make a gravy.

Pour the gravy on each shank and serve with roasted potatoes and a glass or two of dark and stormy ale.

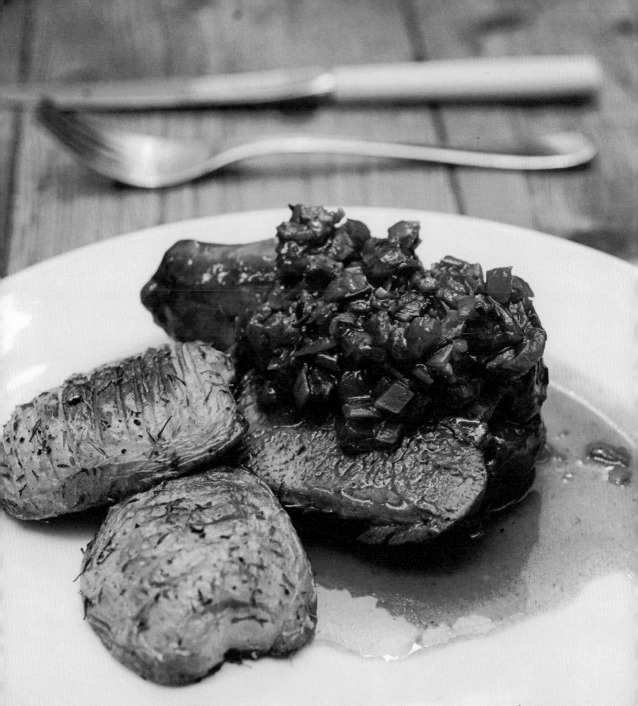

MOST PEOPLE WOULDN'T CONSIDER BEER AS AN INGREDIENT IN COOKING, BUT IT'S WORTH
TRYING JUST FOR THE DIVERSE FLAVORS IT ADDS. THIS DARK AND STORMY SHANKS MEAL
IS A GOOD INTRODUCTION IF YOU HAVEN'T ALREADY USED BEER IN COOKING. THE MORE
I USE BEER IN COOKING THE MORE IT CONFIRMS THAT, JUST LIKE PARMESAN CHEESE,
THE BETTER QUALITY AND MORE COMPLEX THE FLAVOR, THE MORE POSITIVE THE IMPRINT
AN INGREDIENT WILL LEAVE ON THE END PRODUCT. I INITIALLY STARTED USING BEER IN
COOKING WITH MY BOLOGNAISE SAUCE (WHICH IF DISCOVERED, ANY RED BLOODED ITALIAN
WOULD CUT MY HEAD OFF WITH A MEAT CLEAVER). IT BROUGHT A SPECIAL TOUCH TO
THE SAUCE THAT NO ONE COULD FIGURE OUT. I ALSO USED CHILI AND SUGAR IN MY
BOLOGNAISE...CHOP!

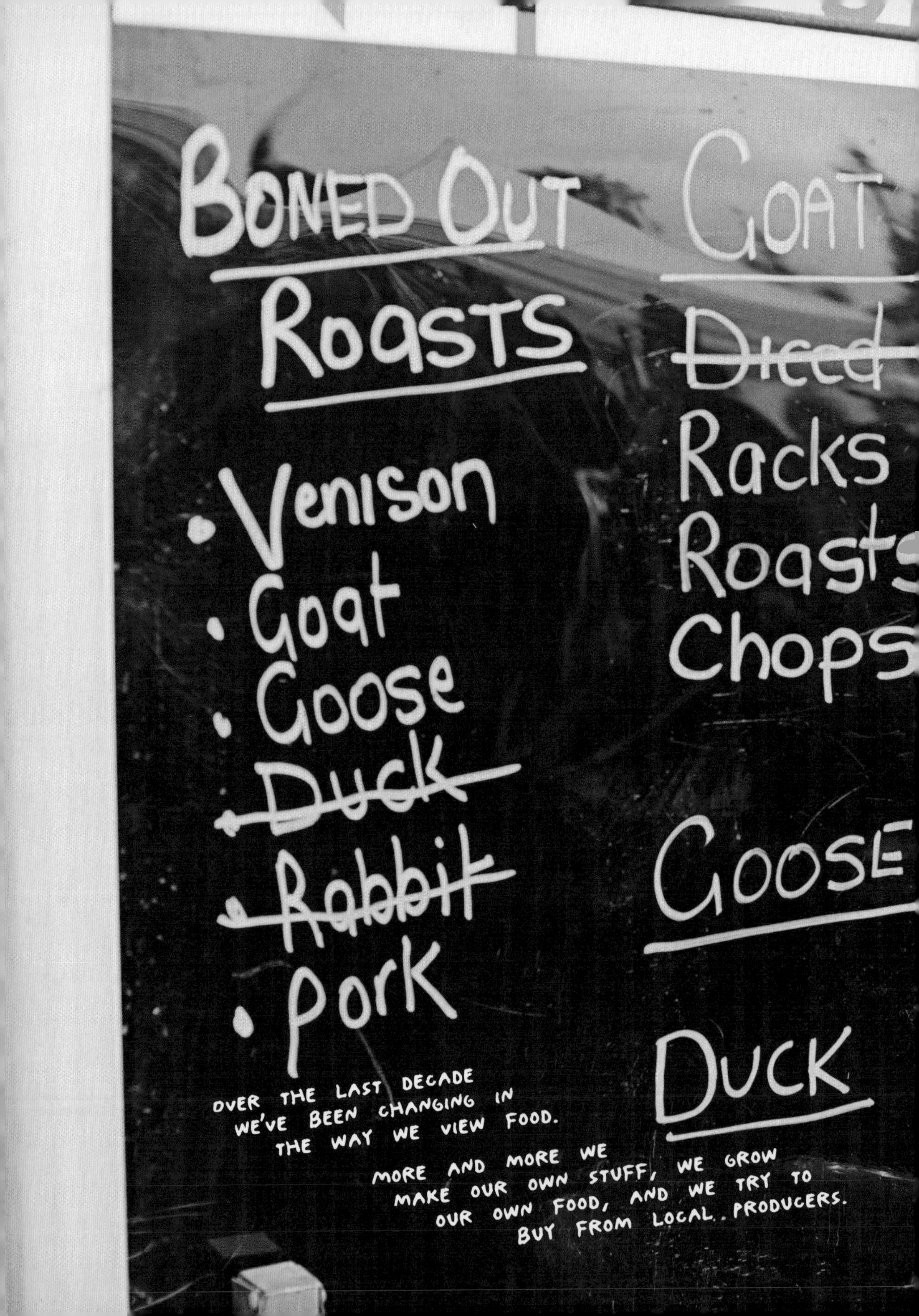

BONED OUT
Roasts

- Venison
- Goat
- Goose
- ~~Duck~~
- ~~Rabbit~~
- Pork

GOAT

~~Diced~~

Racks
Roasts
Chops

GOOSE

DUCK

OVER THE LAST DECADE
WE'VE BEEN CHANGING IN
THE WAY WE VIEW FOOD.

MORE AND MORE WE
MAKE OUR OWN STUFF, WE GROW
OUR OWN FOOD, AND WE TRY TO
BUY FROM LOCAL PRODUCERS.

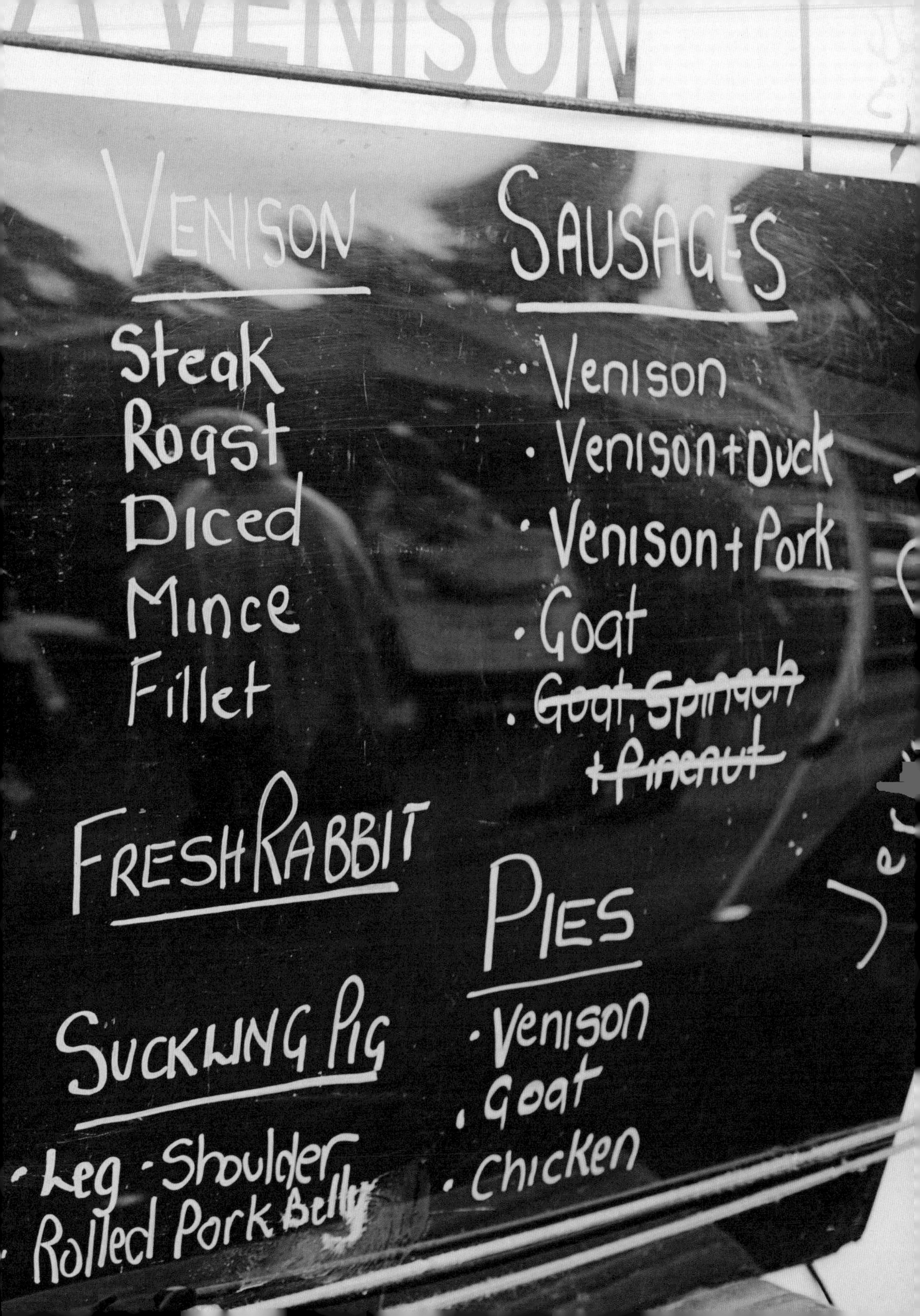

VENISON

VENISON

- Steak
- Roast
- Diced
- Mince
- Fillet

SAUSAGES

- Venison
- Venison+Duck
- Venison+Pork
- Goat
- ~~Goat, Spinach +Pinenut~~

FRESH RABBIT

SUCKLING PIG

- Leg
- Shoulder
- Rolled Pork Belly

PIES

- Venison
- Goat
- Chicken

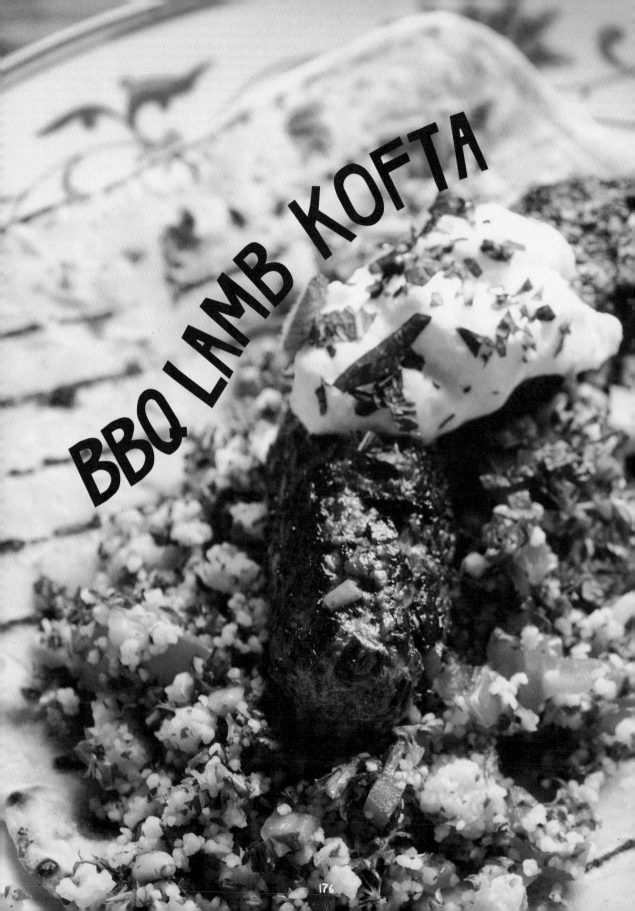

BBQ LAMB KOFTA

I DON'T THINK I EAT ANY MEAT THAT ISN'T ENHANCED BY EITHER SPICES OR HERBS. I FIND A STEAK ON ITS OWN VERY DULL. EVEN LAMB CHOPS NEED SOMETHING, LIKE FRIED SAGE AND PLENTY OF ROSEMARY. IT'S HARDWIRED IN ME TO USE SPICES, OR HERBS—PERSONAL PREFERENCE I SUPPOSE.

A KOFTA TAKES A RELATIVELY BLAND MINCED MEAT AND TURNS IT INTO SOMETHING MORE EXCITING. SERVED WITH THE RIGHT ACCOMPANIMENTS IT CAN BECOME A VERY SIMPLE, YET TASTY TREAT. I LIKE TO COOK MINE ON THE BBQ TO GET THAT SMOKY FLAVOR, BUT YOU CAN FRY THEM INSIDE, AND YOU CAN MAKE IT WITH BEEF, VENISON, OR GOAT IF YOU PREFER.

IF YOU HAVE A BBQ OR WEBBER THAT HAS BOTH A FLAT SURFACE AND A GRILL THEN ONCE YOU HAVE COOKED THE KOFTA ON THE GRIDDLE FOR A FEW MINUTES AND THEY'RE HOLDING THEIR SHAPE WELL, YOU CAN COOK THEM ON THE GRILL WITH SOME BURNING ROSEMARY UNDERNEATH.

WHAT YOU NEED:

Kofta:
1 lb (500 g) minced lamb
1 x egg whisked
2 x cloves fresh garlic, diced
1/2 x red onion, finely diced
1 x fresh chili, diced (or 1/2 tsp of powdered)
Greek yogurt
1/2 cup parsley, finely chopped
1/2 cup mint, finely chopped
1 tsp ground cumin
1 tsp ground coriander
1 tsp cinnamon
1 handful breadcrumbs

Fresh Tabouleh (see page 34)

Turkish Gozleme (Flat Bread):
4 cups plain flour (sifted)
1.5 cups lukewarm water
1/4 cup olive oil
Additional plain flour for dusting
Pinch of salt

HOW TO:

GOZLEME:

First let's make the flat bread. It's the easiest bread ever! Simply mix all the bread ingredients in an electric mixer or by hand, knead for 10 minutes, place in a flour dusted bowl and cover for a an hour.

Roll out with a rolling pin, working your way from the middle out, rub over some olive oil and fold over itself twice and roll out flat again. Repeat this process a few times, and then roll out to a thickness of less than less than 1/4 in (1/2 cm) to form a flat round shape. Grill on the BBQ or griddle pan until crisp on both sides.

KOFTA:

In a large mixing bowl add all the ingredients and mix well using your hands. Go on, get dirty!

Roll out into small sausages.

Place on a flour dusted tray, cover with cling wrap and refrigerate for a few hours, (if possible overnight).

*(optional) Place a few sprigs of rosemary under the BBQ grill but don't turn it on yet.

On the flat BBQ grill heat some olive oil, and start cooking the kofta.

When the kofta will hold their shape, you can place them on the grill (the rosemary will burn and give the kofta a smoky tinge).

Plate the flat bread, spoon over some tabouleh, a lamb kofta, and a dollop of Greek yogurt, then garnish with chopped parsley and mint.

WANT TO GET ALL CARNIVOROUS? EATING RIBS IS ABOUT AS PRIMAL AS IT GETS. IT'S MESSY. IT'S SEXY... WELL MAYBE NOT GLAMOROUS-SEXY BUT IT SURE IS PLENTY OF FUN. I'M FORTUNATE TO BE ABLE TO BUY DIRECT FROM THE GUY THAT RAISES THE PIGS, WHICH SATISFIES ALL MY REQUIREMENTS: HAPPY HOME, ORGANIC, AND A GOOD LIFE, ERGO GOOD END. I ALSO HAVE A MATE THAT KEEPS HIS OWN BEES, WHICH, TO BE HONEST, ISN'T SOMETHING I'M QUITE PREPARED TO DO. GO FIGURE.

THIS IS A MEAL I'LL COOK IN COOLER WEATHER, AND WHEN CONDITIONS ARE RIGHT I'LL USE THE WOOD FIRED OVEN... JUST BECAUSE ITS ACE. AND WHILE IT COOKS YOU CAN SHARE A FEW COLD ALES WITH FRIENDS LISTENING TO THE CRACKLING FIRE AND SUCK UP THE SMELL OF THE SIZZLING RIBS. OH AND IF YOU'RE WONDERING WHAT RO-ATOUILLE IS THEN I SHOULD EXPLAIN. IT'S MY VERSION OF RATATOUILLE. IT'S MAKES GOOD USE OF SOME OF MY FAVORITE SUMMER VEGGIES, AND CUTS THROUGH THE FATTINESS OF A FEED OF RIBS.

WHAT YOU NEED:

The Ribs:
Rack of ribs...
   (they come from pigs)
10 x cloves garlic
1-2 x fresh chili, whole
3 tbsp honey
2 tbsp smoked pimentón
   (Spanish paprika)
A sprig of rosemary
Olive oil

The Ro-Atouille:
1 x large eggplant, chopped
1 x large onion, chopped
2 x small zucchini, chopped
4 x cloves garlic, diced
1 cup of chicken stock
1 cup of dry white wine
1 cup of passata (see page 212)
2 tbsp fresh basil, chopped
2 tbsp dukkah
1 tbsp fresh thyme, chopped
Olive oil
Salt
Pepper

HOW TO:

THE RIBS:

Crush the garlic, chili, and rosemary with a mortar and pestle until you've formed a paste, then add a nice glug of olive oil. Mix well.

Add the pimentón and stir all the flavors through.

Scoop out the mix and add to a small saucepan with the honey, and hold above a gas stove just so you get enough heat into the honey to be able to mix it with the spices and herbs. Mix well.

Rub the marinade over the ribs. All over it baby. It's dirty work but it smells great. No, don't eat the ribs raw—they taste better cooked.

Seal in a container and refrigerate overnight.

To cook, simply wrap the ribs in aluminum foil and bake on a roasting tray in an oven for 30 minutes at around 375-400 F (180-200 C).

THE RO-ATOUILLE:

Heat some olive oil in a frying pan, then add the onion and fry it up until you get some color. Add the chopped eggplant, garlic, and zucchini, and continue to fry giving it a stir regularly.

Add the white wine and cook off until reduced.

Now add the stock and passata and the chopped herbs, and season with salt and pepper. Simmer until all veggies are soft and full of flavor.

Just prior to serving, add the dukkah and stir through. I like to sprinkle some on top when I serve it too. I figure you can never have too much dukkah.

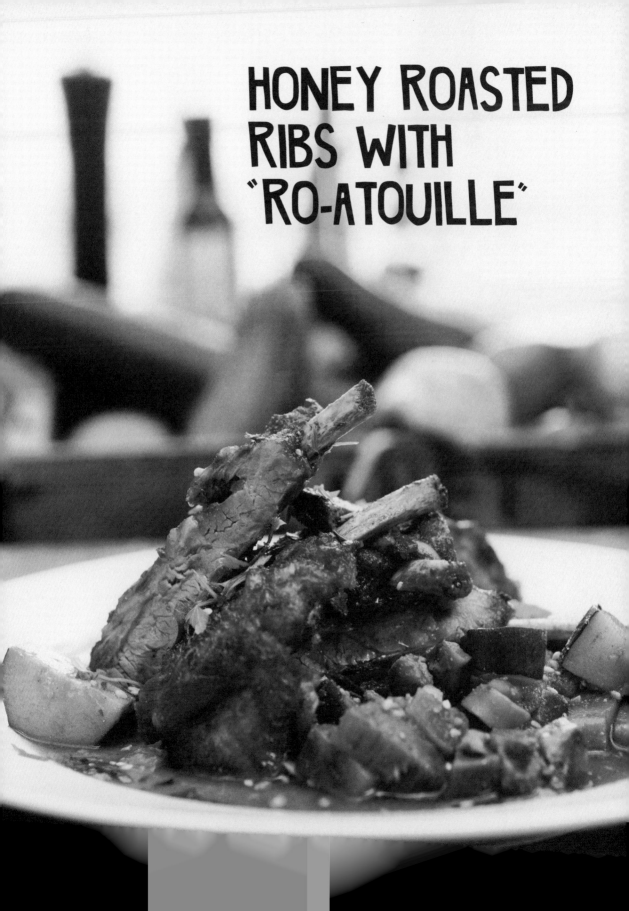

HONEY ROASTED RIBS WITH "RO-ATOUILLE"

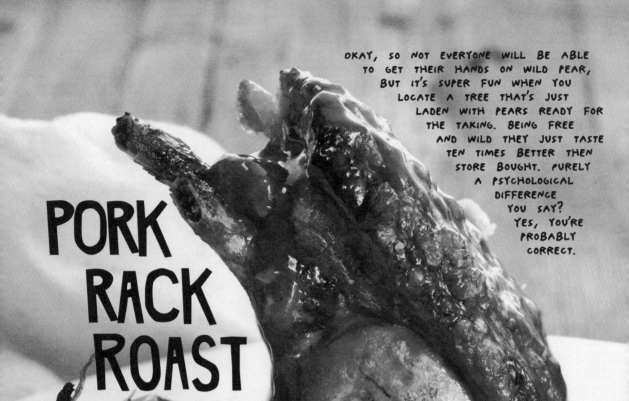

PORK RACK ROAST

OKAY, SO NOT EVERYONE WILL BE ABLE
TO GET THEIR HANDS ON WILD PEAR,
BUT IT'S SUPER FUN WHEN YOU
LOCATE A TREE THAT'S JUST
LADEN WITH PEARS READY FOR
THE TAKING. BEING FREE
AND WILD THEY JUST TASTE
TEN TIMES BETTER THEN
STORE BOUGHT. PURELY
A PSYCHOLOGICAL
DIFFERENCE
YOU SAY?
YES, YOU'RE
PROBABLY
CORRECT.

WITH HONEY-ROASTED WILD PEAR

I SOURCE MOST OF MY PORK FROM THIS LOVELY COUPLE THAT FARM THEIR PIGS WITH THE UTMOST INTEGRITY. THEY HAVE SUCH A GREAT PROCESS; THE PIGS ARE HAPPY, I'M HAPPY. PORK IS ONE OF THE MOST EXCITING MEATS TO ROAST. I MEAN COME ON, WHO DOESN'T LOVE CRACKLING? WELL THE VEGANS AND VEGETARIANS. OH, THEN THERE ARE THE VARIOUS RELIGIONS. WELL I GUESS THEY HAVE NO IDEA WHAT THEY'RE MISSING OUT ON! MORE FOR US, EH?

IF THE PORK IS GOOD QUALITY I DON'T LIKE TO DO ANYTHING TO IT APART FROM SALT FOR THE CRACKLING. NO FLAVORING WHILE ROASTING IS REQUIRED. IT SHOULD BE PERFECT JUST THE WAY IT IS.

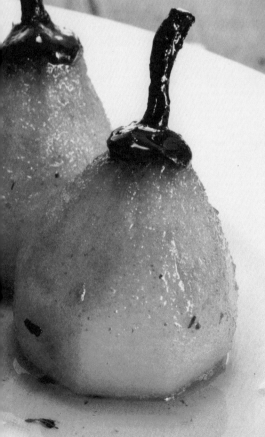

+ GARDEN VEG

WHAT YOU NEED:

1 x pork rack roast with crackling

Pears (if wild they might be small, so maybe 2 per serving)

Mixed garden veg (carrots, potatoes, shallots; whatever is ready and good for roasting)

1 cup water

2 tbsp brown sugar

1 tbsp cinnamon

3 tbsp honey

Cooking salt

HOW TO:

Peel the pears and set in a high-wall baking dish (as the pears will be cooking in hot liquid).

In a saucepan mix the honey, cinnamon, and water, and hold over a flame just enough to melt the honey so you can stir the ingredients. Pour the mix over the pears, and then sprinkle the sugar on top.

Using a very sharp knife cut slits in the crackling and rub with cooking salt.

Roast for 25 minutes on the highest heat your oven will go. Mine tops off at roughly 480 F (250 C). This is important in getting that perfect crackling.

Bake the pears at the same time as the pork (in a separate baking dish).

In another baking dish, toss the garden veg with some chopped herbs, maybe thyme or rosemary, drizzle with olive oil and place in the oven for the last 10 minutes at the high temp.

After the first 25 minutes, reduce heat and roast for another 20 minutes at 340 F (170 C). Take this opportunity to spoon the liquid mix over the pears and return to the oven to finish baking.

When the pork is done, remove and rest while the veg and pears continue to bake until the veg is perfectly roasted (feel free to remove a carrot or two for an official test).

Serve up the pork and veg. When you serve the pears I like to drizzle some of the pear roasting juice over them.

A mouthful of pork and slice of the pear...unbelievable!

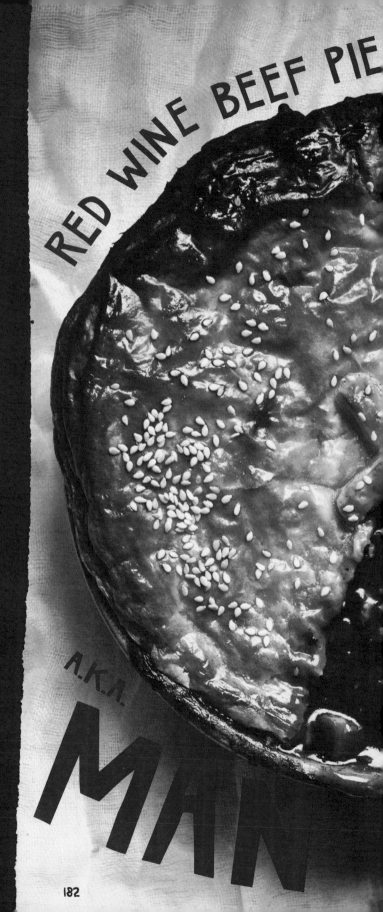

RED WINE BEEF PIE

A.K.A. MAN

T DAWNED ON ME ONE DAY:
WHY USE ONE TYPE OF MEAT
N A PIE WHEN YOU CAN USE
WO? I GUESS THE CARNIVORE
NSIDE GOT THE BETTER OF ME.
F YOU LIKE BEEF BOURGUIGNON
YOU'LL LIKE THIS DISH. IT'S A
VERY HEARTWARMING, COOL-
WEATHER MEAL. SO, LIGHT THE
FIRE, PUT ON A CHET BAKER
ALBUM, OPEN A BOTTLE OF
RED, AND ENJOY.

WHAT YOU NEED:

24 oz (700 g) gravy beef
4 x Italian pork sausages, sliced thick
x egg
Puff pastry (I'm lazy, I buy the pre-made
   version)
2 x onions, chopped
x young leek, chopped
2 x stalks celery, chopped
x carrots, chopped
2 cups mushrooms, chopped
2 x dried chili, chopped
2 x bottles red wine
6 x fresh bay leaves
2 tbsp fresh thyme
tbsp crushed black peppercorn
tbsp corn flower
Butter
Olive oil
Salt
Pepper

HOW TO:

In a large frying pan heat a generous
glug of olive oil. Brown and sear the
beef for a few minutes without cooking
t all the way through. Remove from the
pan and place into a large cast iron or
baked enamel dish. Do the same with
the sausages.

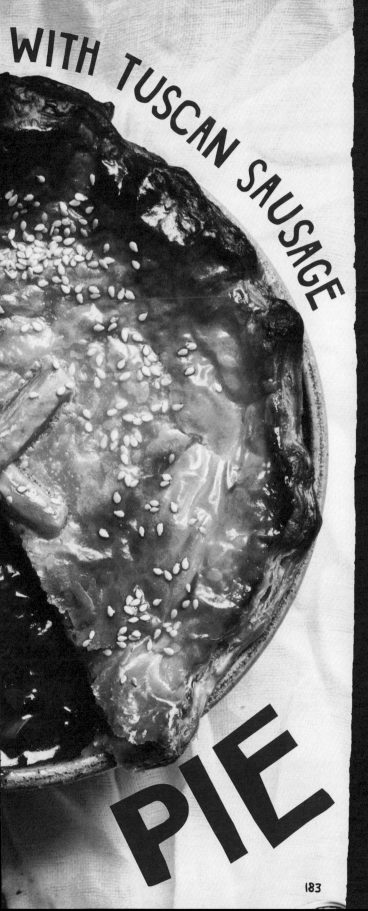

WITH TUSCAN SAUSAGE PIE

Heat a knob of butter in the same pan with a glug of olive oil and sweat the veggies for around 5–10 minutes until you get color.

Transfer to the cast iron dish with the meat. Add the chopped, dried chili. Chili is optional but it does make the dish a bit more interesting.

Deglaze the pan with a half-cup of the red wine. Scrape any flavor off the pan and transfer to the baking dish.

Heat the remaining wine in a saucepan and boil for a few minutes. Then transfer to the baking dish. Mix well, then simmer on a low heat for at least an hour or until the beef is so tender it falls apart when exposed to a blunt spoon. If the sauce is too runny, then mix in a tbsp of corn flower and a little bit of water, stirring well to ensure no lumps remain before you add it to the sauce dish. Stir and simmer with the lid off if you need to reduce it further.

Allow the stew to cool down completely. I even like to store it in a fridge overnight. I'm convinced it allows the flavors to penetrate further.

Spoon out the stew in a pie dish making sure you fill it all the way to the top. Then cover with the puff pastry and push down the pastry to the side of the pie dish with your fingers. Brush with whisked egg and sprinkle over some sesame seeds if you want to make it look fancy.

Bake for 10 minutes at 425 F (220 C) and then a further 10 minutes at 350 F (180 C).

Serve with a smile and maybe a good quality, heavy beer.

WARNING: This dish may encourage growth of hair on upper lip.

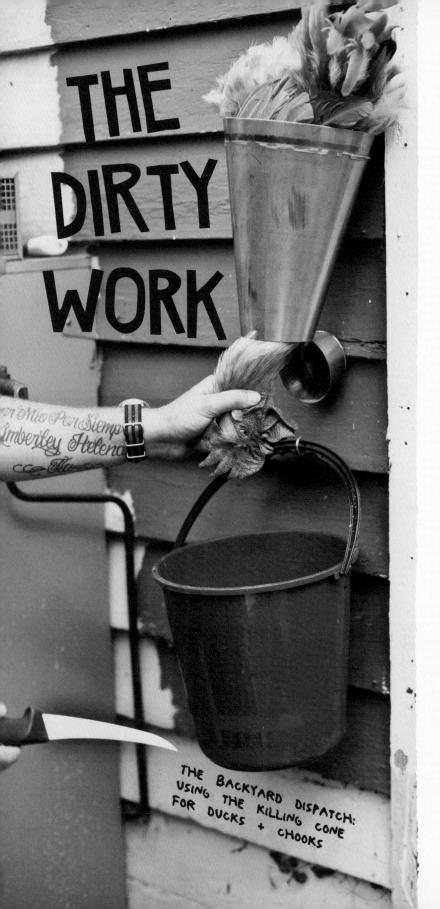

THE DIRTY WORK

THE BACKYARD DISPATCH: USING THE KILLING CONE FOR DUCKS + CHOOKS

Often friends and acquaintances will offer me unwanted birds for me to dispatch and use for meat. It's a great deal, as I don't currently have the space to raise a bunch of ducks and chooks, but I do know how to kill them and prepare their carcasses for cooking.

Now, before I explain how I dispatch birds let me explain the "joys" of home-raised meat. Cooking a two-year-old rooster requires a little more attention than just popping it in an oven and roasting it like a normal store-bought bird. Many older birds are better suited for a braising and then slow cooking in a stew or tagine. There is nothing wrong with the meat, it's just a little tougher, and so it needs special treatment to soften it up. The reason for this is age. Commercial chickens only live for a few months, thus they tend to be more tender...oh that and the fact that they've been bred to be extremely tender and fast growing, and they're not allowed to exercise, and they're fed more food than they need. Don't get me started on commercial chicken production! I think we all know where that's going to go.

Set up a "killing cone" (see image). You can buy these from poultry stores or make one yourself out of something salvaged like I did. Make sure it's securely fastened to the wall/post as the last thing you want in this situation is for your gear to let you down. Before you start the dispatch process make sure you have a large pot of scalding hot water for dipping the bird into pre-feather-plucking. Don't have it boiling, but instead keep it around 150–175 F (70–80 C). Also make sure you have some system to hang the bird once it's dead so you can have hands free to pluck feathers.

Once you have everything set up, you need to get your head in the right place; you need to have you're emotions in check. You are about to take a life with your own capable hands. I have a process that works for me—sure it might seem a little gross, but it's my approach. I play Cuban music through the whole process from start to finish. Why? No, not because I'm some sort of sicko, but because Cuban music makes me happy, and emotionally I need something to distract me from the task at hand. This process never gets easier with time, but I like meat enough to persevere. Do whatever works for you.

It's ultra imperative that you have a razor-sharp knife. If it's not sharp then you're going to make it tough on yourself and obviously the bird. Place the bird head first into the cone and pull out the head through the hole in the bottom of the cone. With the bird sitting upside down gently grab the head and find the jugular on the upper neck of the bird. This is where you need to make a clean slice. In one motion slice the jugular while firmly holding the head and break the bird's neck with a yank. This is a double kill. It ensures that the bird won't suffer for very long. The bird will shake and wobble and blood may get splashed around. This is the bit where most people freak out. It's like when you donk a trout on the head; it's dead straight away, but the nerves in the body still have something to

say. In a few minutes the body will stop wriggling. It's time to move onto the plucking process.

Dip the entire bird into the scalding water for 30 seconds, as this will loosen the feathers and make them very easy to pluck. Hang the bird by its feet and begin to remove the feathers. I tend to have some garbage bags laid directly underneath to collect the wet feathers. I like to start with the hardest feathers to remove while the bird is still hot; these are the tail feathers and the wing feathers. Then I work my way around the entire bird removing all the feathers until only the very fine "pin" hairs remain (these will be burnt off by cooking the bird).

Next you need to remove the innards. Using a sharp knife cut, around the anus/cloaca making sure not to pierce internal organs as this can spoil the meat and the experience. I tend to cut a circle starting underneath the cloaca up to just below the breast cavity and back again. This will make sense when you have a naked bird in your hands. Pull out all the organs, setting aside the heart and liver if you intend to use these for further cooking. Chicken liver makes amazingly good pate. Ensure you pull out everything, and you will need to dig out the lungs as they kind of hide in the chest cavity. Cut out the anus and rinse the inside of the bird and hang to dry. If you have a heat-sealing Cryovac, seal up the bird when it is dry, pop it in the freezer, and the job is done. You've just done something that most people don't want to think about, even though they're quite happy to devour a chicken burger. Well done!

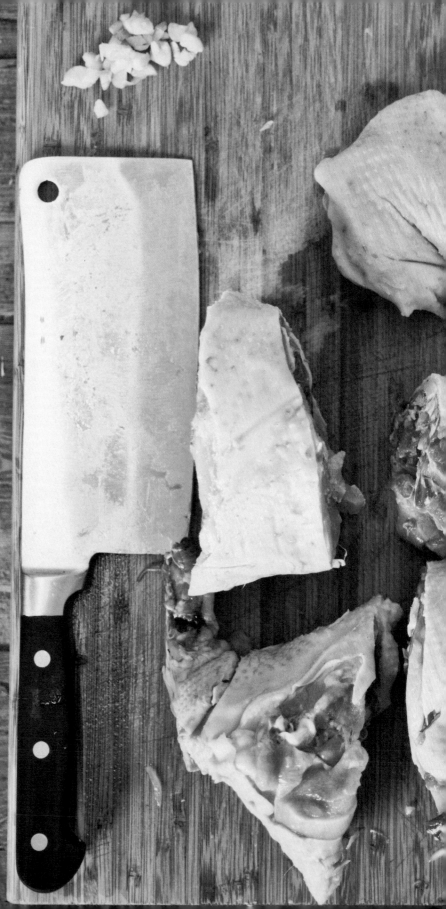

I'VE ALWAYS SAID THAT IT'S A PRIVILEGE FOR US TO EAT MEAT, AND IF YOU HONESTLY CAN'T BRING YOURSELF TO "ACQUIRE" YOUR OWN MEAT, THEN YOU SHOULDN'T EAT IT.

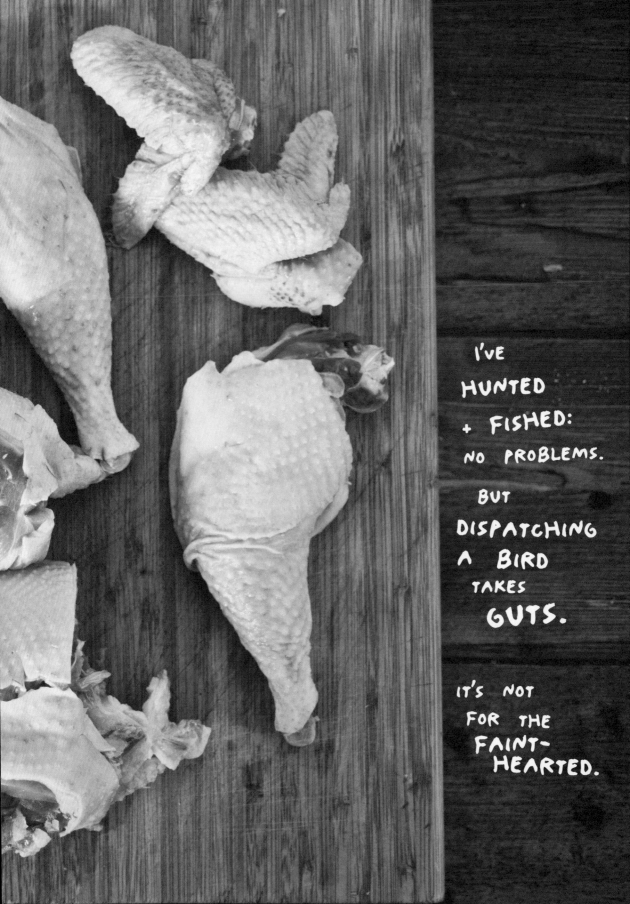

I'VE
HUNTED
+ FISHED:
NO PROBLEMS.

BUT
DISPATCHING
A BIRD
TAKES
GUTS.

IT'S NOT
FOR THE
FAINT-
HEARTED.

I KNOW. IT SOUNDS EXCESSIVE WRAPPING ONE MEAT WITH ANOTHER, BUT HECK. THESE ANIMALS GAVE US THEIR LIVES, THE LEAST WE CAN DO IS TREAT THEM WITH RESPECT BY MAKING THEM AS DELICIOUS AS POSSIBLE! WE CURE OUR OWN JAMÓN EVERY YEAR (SEE PAGE 216) AND IT'S A GREAT TREAT. IT IS SO FULL OF FLAVOR THAT IT TURNS THE EXCITEMENT LEVEL OF THIS DISH ALL THE WAY UP TO 11. SO WHEN I GET THE PHONE CALL FROM SOMEONE OFFERING ME THEIR CHOOKS TO DISPATCH I WILL OFTEN HAVE THIS DISH IN MIND. IF YOU'RE NOT SURE HOW TO CUT OUT THE THIGH FROM A COMPLETE BIRD THERE ARE INSTRUCTIONAL VIDEOS ONLINE... ALONGSIDE SOME OTHER PRETTY WEIRD SHIT, LET'S BE HONEST.

THE SIDE SALAD ISN'T ALL ROASTED BUT IT SOUNDS GOOD THAT WAY. WITH THE CAPSICUM AND EGGPLANT I TEND TO COOK A FEW AT A TIME, THEN USE WHAT I NEED FOR THIS DISH AND STORE THE REST IN THE FRIDGE FOR ANOTHER TIME.

JAMÓN-WRAPPED CHICKEN WITH ROASTED SUMMER VEG SALAD

HOW TO:
THE CHICKEN:

Mix the pesto and ricotta in a bowl.

Spoon some of the cheese/pesto mix on the inside of the thigh, then wrap and roll up the thigh fillet with a slice of jamón. You can use a wooden skewer to hold it all together or just lay them closely together on the baking tray. Feel free to use more than one slice of jamón per fillet. Drizzle with olive oil.

Bake for 25 minutes at 400 F (200 C).

THE ROAST SALAD:

Bake the capsicum at 400 F (200 C) until the skin starts to blacken. Don't panic, this is what we want to happen.

When it's done, remove and place in a plastic bag to cool. Seal well.

At the same time you bake the capsicum, bake the cherry tomatoes (sliced in half) with a good drizzle of magic olive oil for 25 minutes.

Slice the eggplant lengthwise and grill on a hot griddle pan with a dash of oil on each slice. This takes a while, so it's nice to have a cold glass of wine close-by to keep you company. When all the slices are nicely grilled set aside to cool.

Mix the cooked veg in a bowl, add the red wine vinegar, the regular feta, and also the parsley, but not the marinated goats' feta just yet. Season to taste with salt and pepper.

Dish up the chicken along with the roast veg. Garnish each plate with a few spoonfuls of the goats' feta and finish off with a sprinkle of pine nuts.

WHAT YOU NEED:

The Chicken:
6 x chicken thighs
6 x slices of jamón thinly sliced
   (you can sub prosciutto)
9 oz (250 g) ricotta
3 tbsp pesto (see page 208)

The Salad:
1 x eggplant
1 x large, red capsicum
Cherry tomatoes
1.75 oz (50 g) feta
Marinated goats' feta (garnish)
2 x tbsp red wine vinegar
1 x tbsp parsley, finely chopped
Pine nuts
Olive oil
Salt
Pepper

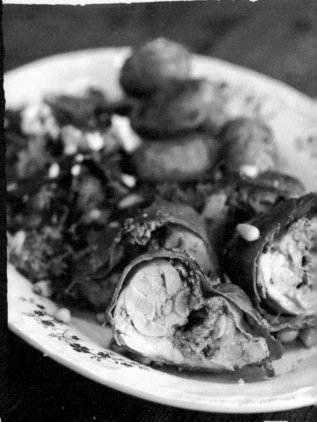

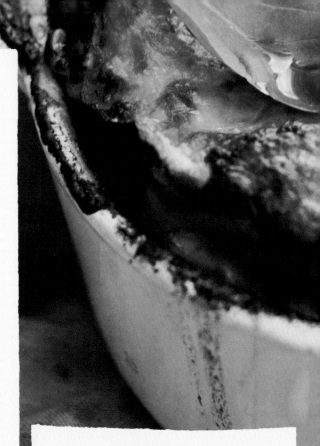

HOW TO:

Slice the eggplant lengthwise and grill on a griddle pan with a generous splash of olive oil for each slice. When done set aside to cool.

In a large pot, heat some olive oil and brown the chicken pieces for a few minutes on each side, but don't cook them through. Once done, set aside.

In the same pot, heat some olive oil and add the onions, carrots, and celery. Cook for a good while until they are softened and have changed color.

Now add the wine and cook out.

When the wine is almost all cooked out return the chicken, and add the passata and garlic.

Cook until the meat falls from the bone. Depending on the age and type of bird this will take from 40–60 minutes

Remove the pieces of chicken and scrape the meat off the bone. Return the meat to the pot and discard the bones.

Now add the basil.

Allow the chicken mix to cool to room temp.

At the same time cook the lasagna pasta al dente.

Preheat the oven to 400 F (200 C).

In a large bowl stir the ricotta, cheddar, and Parmesan until completely mixed.

Using a large baking dish, ladle out a layer of the chicken ragu, then a layer of grilled eggplant, then lasagna, then cheese. Repeat this process for at least 3 levels.

On top of the last layer grate over plenty of cheddar and parmesan cheese and sprinkle over some pines nuts.

Bake covered with a lid or aluminum foil for 30 minutes then remove the cover and bake for another 20 minutes or until golden brown up top.

WHAT YOU NEED:

1 x whole chicken, quartered (if you don't know how to do this then get your local butcher to do it for you)
1 box lasagna pasta
2 x carrots, finely chopped
2 x celery stalks, finely chopped
3 x eggplants
2 x onions, finely chopped
4 x cloves garlic, finely chopped
1 large handful basil, chopped
2 cups cheddar cheese, grated
2 cups Parmesan cheese, grated
20 oz (600 g) ricotta cheese
24 oz (750 ml) passata (or a tin of chopped tomatoes)
1 cup dry white wine
Pine nuts
Olive oil
Salt
Pepper

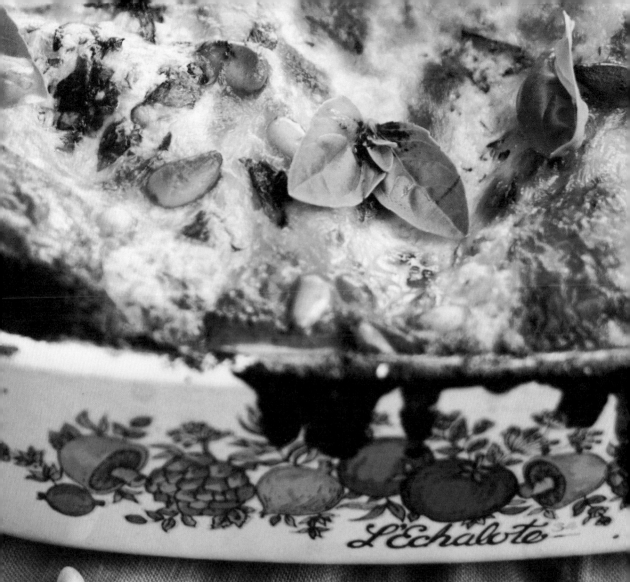

ROAST CHICKEN + GRILLED EGGPLANT LASAGNA

RAISING POULTRY IS NOT A HARD TASK... WELL APART FROM SETTING UP THE CHOOK SHED AND MAKING THE BIRDS COMFORTABLE. BUT WHEN THAT'S BEEN DONE ALL YOU NEED TO DO IS KEEP THEM HAPPILY FED, PROVIDE THEM WATER, AND GIVE THEM SPACE TO RUN AROUND LIKE CHOOKS DO.

A FRIEND OF MINE RAISES HER OWN CHICKENS FROM FERTILIZED EGGS EACH SPRING. SHE HAS ONE OF THOSE BASIC INCUBATORS AND IT'S A BIT OF A LUCKY DIP REALLY: SOME WORK, SOME DON'T HATCH, AND SOME GROW UP TO BE MALES—AND NO ONE WANTS ROOSTERS...

WELL APART FROM ME. IN THE COMMERCIAL POULTRY INDUSTRY MALES ARE DISCARDED IN THE MOST HORRID WAY. IF THEY WERE ALLOWED TO MATURE, THEY'D BE AN EXCELLENT SOURCE OF MEAT. THANKFULLY FOR ME I GET THE UNWANTED BIRDS. ROOSTERS ARE A DIFFERENT BALL GAME FROM 10-WEEK-OLD, SUCCULENT BREED HENS, SO THEY REQUIRE A BIT OF EXTRA CULINARY ATTENTION. TREAT THEM LIKE WILD GAME; BRAISING THEM IS THE BEST APPROACH. BUT IF YOU DON'T HAVE ACCESS TO FREE, YOUNG ROOSTERS THEN USE ETHICALLY SOURCED CHICKENS (I.E. FREE-RANGE ORGANIC IF POSSIBLE). BUT IT'S YOUR CHOICE. IT'S ALWAYS YOUR CHOICE.

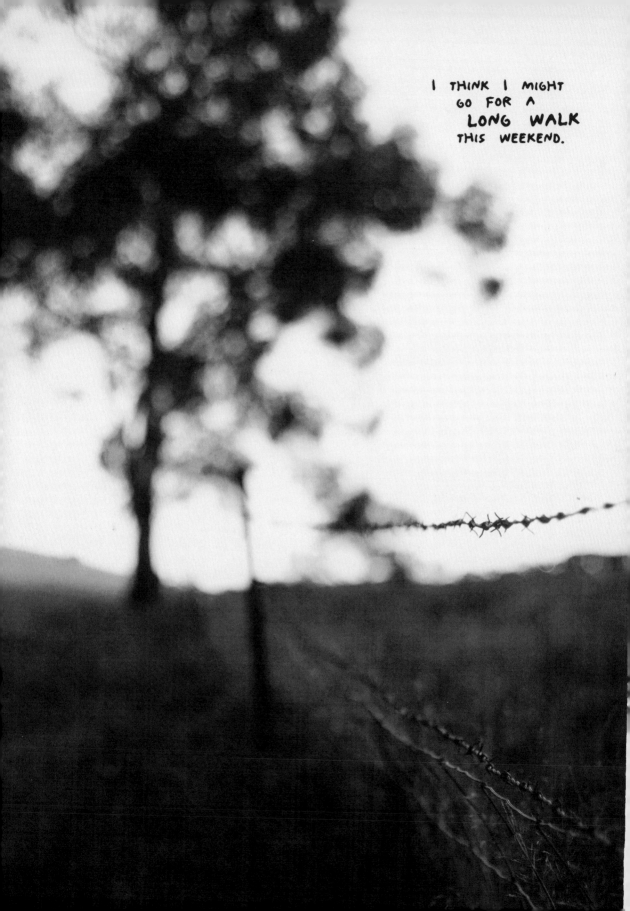

I THINK I MIGHT
GO FOR A
LONG WALK
THIS WEEKEND.

HONEY CHORIZO

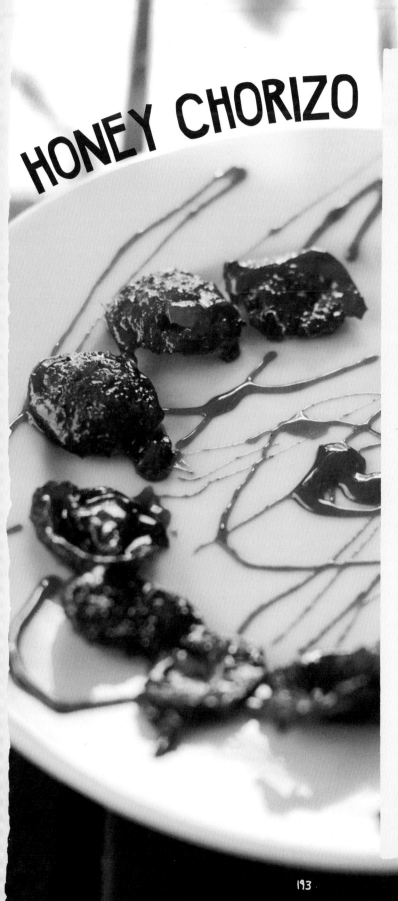

I HAVE A SOFT SPOT FOR THIS TAPA. I HAD ONE OF THOSE SPECIAL FOOD MOMENTS WHILE VISITING NYC TO PHOTOGRAPH A WEDDING FOR SOME FRIENDS OF MINE. WE WERE IN A TAPAS BAR ON A STINKING HOT NEW YORK SUMMER'S DAY DEVOURING BOWLS OF THIS TAPA AND DRINKING SANGRIA BY THE BUCKET LOAD. WHEN WE NEXT CAUGHT UP, I MADE IT AS A SPECIAL TREAT AND NOW EVERY TIME I MAKE IT THE MEMORIES COME STRAIGHT BACK. IT'S FUNNY HOW FOOD DOES THAT.

LIKE MOST OF MY FAVORITE TAPAS, IT'S EASY TO MAKE AND VERY STRONG IN FLAVOR SO YOU WON'T NEED MUCH. WELL, ACTUALLY, I LIE—THAT DEPENDS ON HOW MUCH SANGRIA YOU'VE DRANK.

WHAT YOU NEED:

2 x chorizo sausage
2 x tbsp of your favorite honey
1/2 tsp paprika
1/2 tsp cumin seeds
Olive oil

HOW TO:

Cut the chorizo into slices around 1/2 in (1 cm) thick.

In a mixing bowl, mix the honey, chorizo, and spices.

Panfry in olive oil until crisp (5–10 minutes).

Serve all fancy like, and don't waste that melted honey; spread it around and make pretty patterns.

WLL
BURGER

I CAN'T DENY THAT I'M A SUCKER FOR A GOOD BURGER. AND IT'S NOT SOMETHING THAT I'LL EVER GIVE UP. BUT INSTEAD OF RELYING ON SOME MULTINATIONAL COMPANY TO ACCOMMODATE MY BASIC BURGER DESIRE I LIKE TO MAKE MY OWN. AND I GET TO USE A FEW INGREDIENTS THAT I MAKE MYSELF, NOTABLY THE DILL-PICKLED CUCUMBER, THE KASUNDI, AND SOME FRESH LEEKS FROM THE GARDEN FRIED IN BUTTER AND OLIVE OIL.

WHEN IT COMES TO THE BEEF, I LIKE IT LOCAL AND JUST AS IT COMES. NO EXTRA FLAVOR ADDED, NO BREAD CRUMBS, NO EGGS, JUST PURE, GOOD BEEF. IF THE BEEF IS GOOD QUALITY THEN THE FLAVORS SHOULD SPEAK FOR THEMSELVES. MY BUTCHER ASKS HOW LEAN I WANT THE MIX. SPEAK TO YOUR BUTCHER AND TAKE ADVANTAGE OF THIS OPTION IF AVAILABLE. I LIKE MINE SOMEWHERE BETWEEN SUPER LEAN AND FULL FAT. IT HELPS ME SLEEP AT NIGHT.

WHAT YOU NEED:

18 oz (500 g) beautiful minced beef

Turkish rolls (or burger buns)

1 x leek, sliced

WLL dill-pickled cucumber (see page 226)

WLL kasundi (see page 224)

1.75 oz (50 g) knob of butter

Swiss cheese

Olive oil

Salt

Pepper

HOW TO:

Heat a knob of butter and some olive oil and panfry the sliced leek to your liking. I don't mind it still a bit green, not too burnt. If you don't like leek you can substitute with onions; what we're after is the sweetness of onion. When done, set aside.

Form some patties with the minced beef. I tend to go for thick and bulky, but you can go thin if you like. I figure if you're going to eat a bit of beef you might as well be indulgent!

In the same pan that you fried the leek, heat up some olive oil and fry the burger patties, flipping occasionally.

While the burger is frying slop some hot kasundi on the base of the bun (you can use any relish really but I like the heat of the chili in the kasundi).

When the burger is almost done, pop some slices of Swiss cheese on top, to melt for a minute or so.

Serve the burger on the bun, topped with a few slices of dill cucumber and the fried, buttery leek goodness.

Add a bit of salt and pepper, and wash down with a cold beer (cold beer is optional but highly recommended).

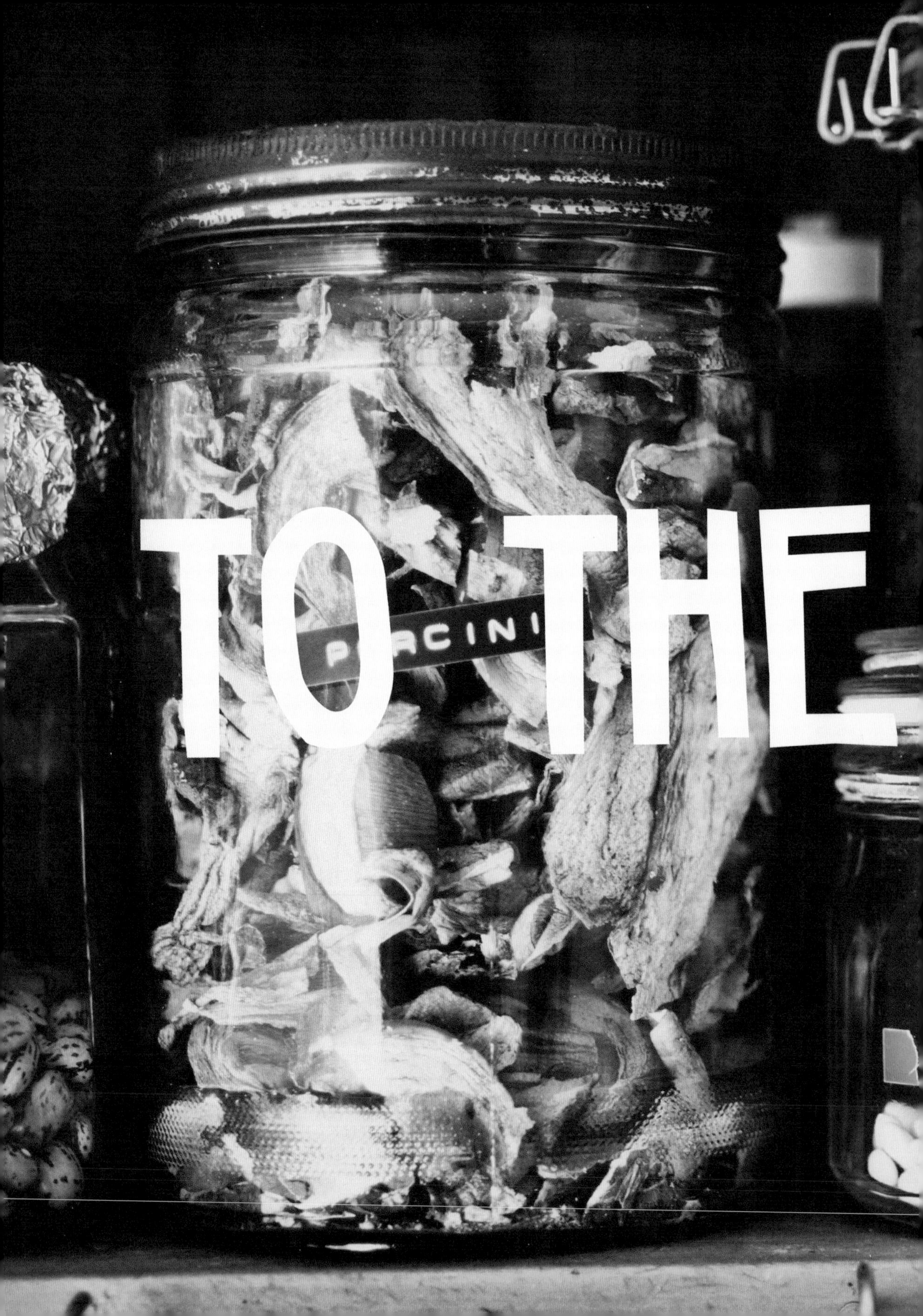

TO THE

LARDER

Tomato
Relish

CANNELLINI

PINE NUTS

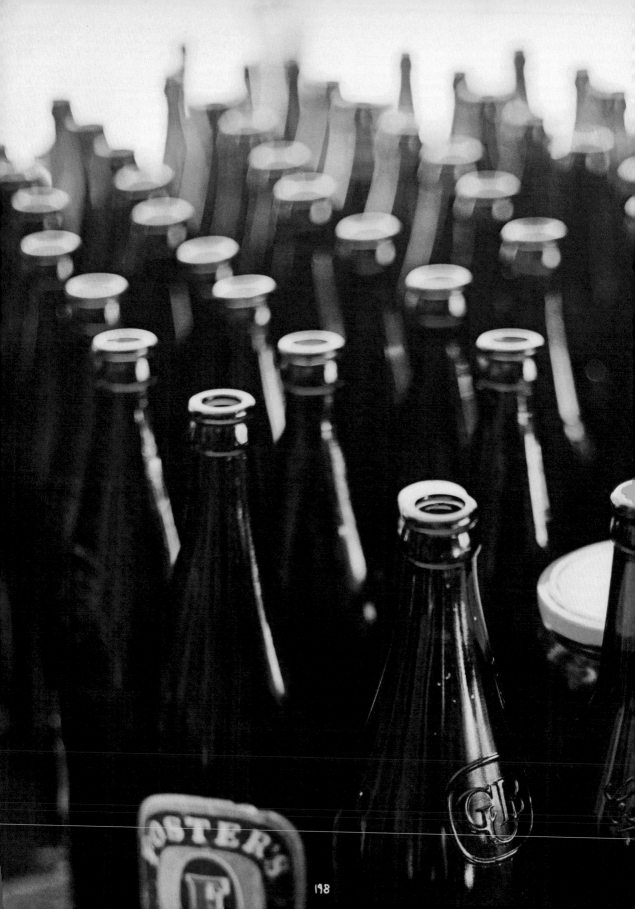

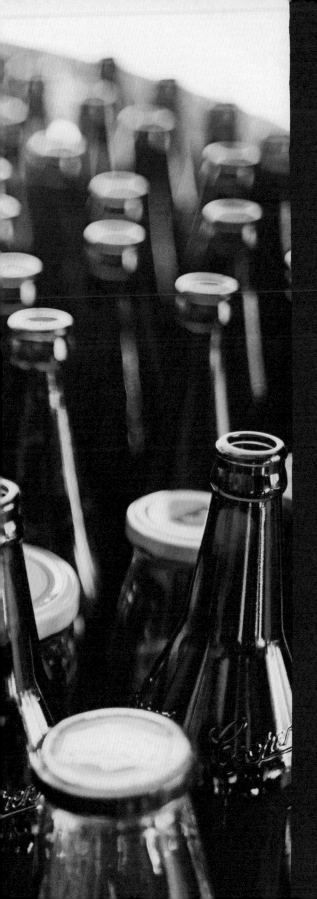

There's nothing new about the concept of a larder. People have been keeping stores for centuries. The difference now is that most of our pantries are full of food that we've had no hand in producing. Instead it's all being bought at the supermarket. Unfortunately for us they can often be some pretty dodgy foods, with many being highly processed and full of food additives, artificial flavor enhancers, and plenty of excess sodium and sugars. All these unnatural ingredients are "necessary" to keep the food in whatever state has been determined to be the most marketable and fiscally prudent. However, in days gone by, people would use traditional methods to store some of what they grew during the warmer months so they would have a reliable food supply over the cooler months. How did these people survive without supermarkets?

Out of this necessity to store food have come some of our favorite foods: dried, cured sausages and ham come to mind; then there are smoked goods; pickles; jams; relish; chutney; jellies; and cheeses. There are so many members of the larder club that one could spend a lifetime researching all the possibilities and never have a complete list. I've outlined a few of the basics, so you can just dip your toe in the water, so to speak.

It should be mentioned that this section works in correlation with, and as a sort of solution to, growing your own food. However, if you don't have the veggie patch, an orchard, or a mature olive grove, then you can rely on alternatives like local markets and produce...and especially, befriending people who do grow their own. For example, I don't own an olive grove but I spend a day laboring away picking olives for a friend, so that in return I get some olives and fresh-pressed, extra-virgin olive oil. I wish the community at large embraced this system, wherein we could help each other in return for goods and services.

HOT ZUCCHINI RELISH

NEAR THE END OF SUMMER, I OFTEN TELL MYSELF I MUST PLANT LESS ZUCCHINI NEXT YEAR, BUT WHEN THE TIME COMES I ALWAYS SEEM TO PLANT MORE. ZUCCHINI IS A WONDERFUL VEGETABLE TO GROW, AS IT DOESN'T REQUIRE MUCH WORK, THE SEEDS ARE EASY TO RAISE, AND THE ZUCCHINI ITSELF TASTES GREAT IN SO MANY FORMS. YOU CAN EVEN EAT THE FLOWERS STUFFED AND FRIED IN BATTER. WHEN YOU HAVE A GLUT OF THIS LOVELY VEGETABLE, OR JUST WANT SOMETHING TO TOP YOUR HOT DOG, BURGER, OR TOASTED SANDWICH THEN THIS IS PERFECT. A GOOD MIX OF SWEET, SOUR, AND HEAT.

THESE MEASUREMENTS ARE A BASE. IF YOU HAVE DOUBLE THE AMOUNT OF ZUCCHINI THEN DOUBLE THE AMOUNT OF EVERYTHING. SAVVY?

WHAT YOU NEED:

6 cups zucchini, chopped (any
   variety, hopefully home grown)
2 x onions
3 x fresh chilies
1/2 x green capsicum
1/2 x red capsicum
1/2 x yellow capsicum
1.5 cups sugar
2 cups vinegar
2 tbsp salt
1 tbsp paprika
2 tsp mustard seed
1 tsp turmeric
1 tsp ground cumin
Olive oil

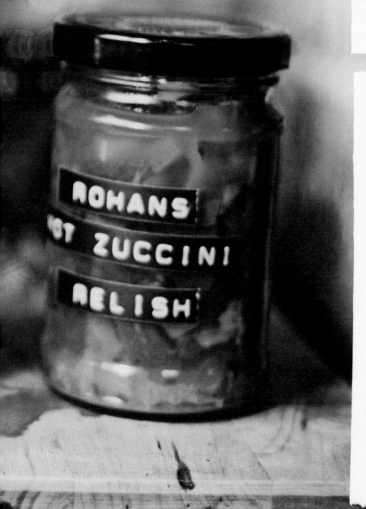

HOW TO:

Chop the vegetables (somewhere between rough and fine).

Place the veggies (except for the chili) in a large mixing bowl and cover with salt. Mix well and let it sit overnight.

In the morning, drain the liquid that has formed from the bowl. Don't drink it.

Heat olive oil in a large saucepan, add the drained vegetables and cook stirring often for at least 10 minutes. This process will soften the veg.

When the veg is cooked through, add the sugar, vinegar, spices, and finely chopped chili. Stir well and simmer for 30 minutes.

Decant in to sterilized jars and label "See, I Can Make Relish."

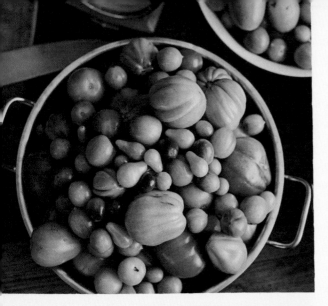

EVERY FEW SUMMERS WE GET DUPED. SOMETIMES THERE JUST AREN'T ENOUGH HOT, SUNNY DAYS NO MATTER HOW MANY COLD BEERS YOU DRINK. ONE YEAR WE ENDED UP WITH LOADS OF GREEN AND SEMI RIPE TOMATOES, AND WE TRIED EVERY TRICK IN THE BOOK TO ARTIFICIALLY OR NATURALLY RIPEN THEM. A FEW METHODS WE TRIED WERE UPROOTING AND HANGING THE ENTIRE PLANT UPSIDE DOWN, LAYING BANANA PEELS AT THE BASE OF THE PLANT, AND FINALLY, THE LEAST SUCCESSFUL METHOD, ASKING THEM (VERY STERNLY) TO RIPEN.

SO, INSTEAD OF DUMPING THEM IN THE COMPOST I STARTED MAKING A RELISH WITH THEM. I STILL PREFER TALKING TO THEM STERNLY NO MATTER HOW INEFFECTIVE.

WHAT YOU NEED:

5.5 lb (2.5 kg) green (and semi ripe) mixed tomatoes
2.75 lb (1.5 kg) onions, diced
5 x green chilies (fresh & including seeds)
2 cups malt vinegar
1.5 cups sugar
2-3 tbsp salt
2 tbsp curry powder
1 tbsp mustard seeds
1 tbsp chili powder
1 tbsp cumin powder

HOW TO:

Finely slice the tomato and onion and place into a large saucepan.

Sprinkle half the salt over them and toss and mix well. Pour over the remaining salt and mix well. Cover and let sit overnight.

The following day drain the excess liquid that has collected in the pan.

Pop the saucepan on the stove and add all the remaining ingredients. Bring to a boil then simmer for an hour.

Store in sanitized jars.

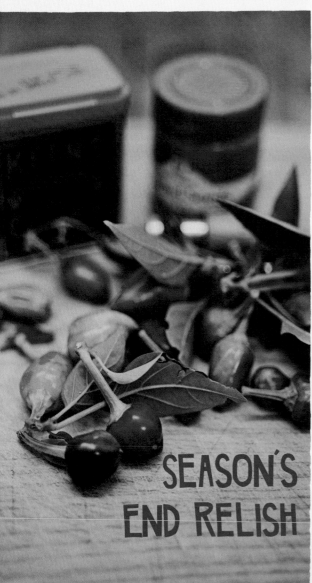

SEASON'S END RELISH

MUM'S TOMATO RELISH

A FEW YEARS AGO WE PAINTED THE OUTSIDE OF OUR HOUSE. ON ONE OF THOSE PAINTING DAYS WE GOT FISH AND CHIPS FOR THE GUYS HELPING US, AND NOT HAVING ANY KETCHUP IN THE PANTRY WE SERVED IT WITH MY MUM'S RELISH INSTEAD. ONE OF THE GUYS LIKED IT SO MUCH HE LATER ASKED FOR MUM'S RECIPE!

NOT HAVING IT MYSELF I REALIZED THAT IT WOULD BE LOST IF I DIDN'T MAKE A RECORD OF IT. SO, AFTER SOME SUAVE COAXING, I EVENTUALLY GOT IT OFF MUM. IT WAS JUST LIKE THE TIME I CONVINCED HER TO GIVE ME HER SPARE COPY OF THE COUNTRY WOMEN'S ASSOCIATION COOKBOOK, WHICH IS FULL OF OLD-TIME COUNTRY RECIPES. TOTAL SCORE!

WHAT YOU NEED:

4 lb mixed tomatoes
2 lb onions, sliced
16 oz (1 pint) malt vinegar
1 cup sugar
3 tbsp salt
1.5 tbsp curry powder
1 tbsp mustard powder
2 tbsp cornflour
Chili powder (optional)

HOW TO:

In boiling hot water scald 4 lb tomatoes. Remove, and skin them.

Chop up the tomatoes and the onions.

Place the tomatoes and onions in separate bowls, sprinkle with a generous amount of salt and leave overnight. Drain excess liquid in the morning.

Boil the onions in a pint of vinegar for 15 minutes.

Add tomatoes with good cup sugar. Mix in the mustard, curry powder, a little cold vinegar, and the cornflour. Boil for 20–30 minutes, stirring in all ingredients. Add a little cayenne or chili powder as preferred.

Use a stick blender to for a quick whiz. Taste and take this opportunity to add extra spices if you see fit... I tend to add more chili at this stage.

Store in sanitized jars.

Serve with fish and chips (optional).

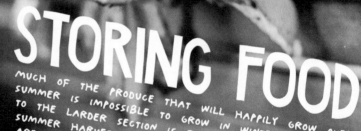

STORING FOOD

MUCH OF THE PRODUCE THAT WILL HAPPILY GROW OVER SUMMER IS IMPOSSIBLE TO GROW IN WINTER. THE STRAIGHT TO THE LARDER SECTION IS FULL OF WAYS TO PRESERVE THE SUMMER HARVEST FOR A WINTER CONSUMPTION. SOME THINGS ARE SO BASIC THEY DON'T REQUIRE A RECIPE PAGE THEMSELVES BUT THEY'RE WORTH A MENTION. SO HERE IS A HANDFUL OF ITEMS THAT MIGHT GET YOU STARTED.

OLIVE OIL:

If you go to the backbreaking effort of picking olives for a day to send them off to be cold pressed then this little bit of information may save you some heartache. Sunlight can turn olive oil into a real mess, so store your olive oil in the dark. Use dark glass if possible. I use tinted wine bottles but you can buy completely sealed bottles made especially for this purpose. I then store them in the darkest spot of my larder with a blanket over them.

BORLOTTI AND CANNELLINI BEANS:

The best way to dry these beans out is to leave them on the vine in the bean pod until autumn. By then, they will have dried up nicely and will look very shriveled. To tell if they're dried properly, shake them, and if they rattle like a maraca open the pod up. Inside, the beans should look like small birds' eggs, and be totally dry. If they aren't firm, leave the beans on the vine for a few weeks longer. Whatever you do, don't remove fresh beans from the pod to dry them, as they tend to dry too quickly and shrivel.

To eat them in winter, soak the dried beans in cold water overnight. Then boil them for 30 minutes or until they're soft enough to add to whatever you're cooking.

PUMPKIN

Pumpkin is one of my favorite things to eat in winter. In soups, gnocchi, roasted, whatever you desire. They keys to successfully storing a pumpkin in the larder are leaving 6 inches (15 cm) of the stalk connected and not removing the pumpkin from the vine until the vine is totally dead and all the leaves have fallen off. If you have a bit of sunny weather on the radar after they have been harvested, you can lay out your pumpkins in the sun for a week or so outside, turning them occasionally. This will also help improve longevity over winter.

WILD MUSHROOMS (DRIED)

If you have a food dehydrator then use it, following the operating instructions. If you're old school like me and don't want another large machine clogging up your kitchen, then use the following method. Clean the mushrooms with a paper towel or small brush and slice them up. Thread fishing line through the sliced mushrooms using a sewing needle. Hang the mushrooms with each end of the fishing line attached in a horizontal line for at least 8 weeks, until crisp and dry. They can be stored in Cryovac bags or in sealed glass jars. But make sure they are completely dried out or they might go bad.

STORING SPUDS (POTATOES)

The best time to plant potatoes is just after the last spring frost. The best time to pick potatoes is when the vegetation that's above ground goes to flower and seed.

I tend to grow potatoes in summer especially for winter consumption as well as growing enough for our summer needs. I'll fill a large bag, which seems to be enough for a family of four. We store ours in the dark, in a spot that is safe from mice and is nice and cool. Before we put the spuds in the bag we'll lay them out (turning occasionally) on a brick path for a few days in the sunlight to "cure." We don't wash the potatoes, as this helps to seal them for storage. We wait until we take them out for cooking to wash them. And just as the bag is almost finished I'll start to plant the spuds that have spouted because it's usually spring by the time the bag is getting near empty.

The key to storing potatoes and getting the most longevity is breathable darkness. If you ever see a real natural-fiber hessian bag, buy it immediately or steal it. There is a reason these are used for potatoes; they're made from natural fibers that are much more breathable than their plastic counterparts. Plastic tends to make the spuds sweat and then rot. Some commercial spud bags can hold up to 90 lb (40 kg)

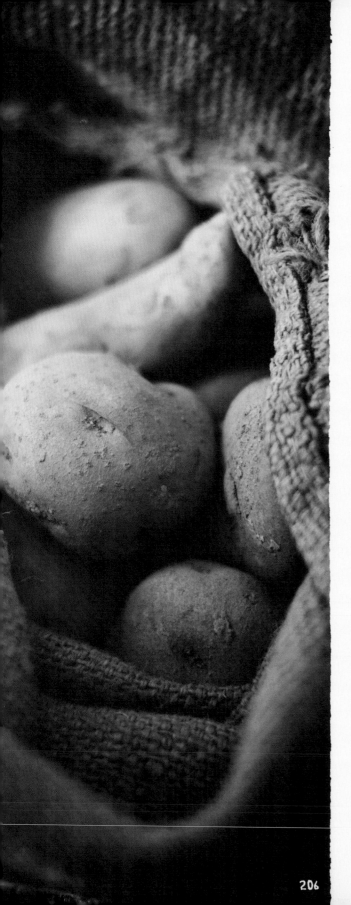

or more. So remember when you fill them up that they might become very heavy to lift. It can become a two-person job to move a filled bag, so if possible, fill it where it will end up being stored.

GARLIC/ONION

If you let the garlic to go to seed in your garden, cut off the pretty, round seed heads as they start to open up and place in a glass jar with no lid. These will dry and become a lovely garnish or you can use them as seeds for next season's crop.

Pull the garlic/onion from the soil when the top part of the plant (that is the bit above the soil) is drying out, turning yellow, and dying off. This is when the garlic is at its peak. Don't cut the stems off. Use jute twine and tie up a bundle of garlic/onion by the stems. Hang it in the hot sun for a week or so, turning every few days to cure. Then hang them off a brick wall where it's dry and free from moisture.

The garlic will store this way for most of the winter, but by late winter some might start to shoot again, which is a good time to pop the individual cloves back in the ground. If you find yourself in the middle of the winter with plenty left to see you through to spring, then use the larger garlic's remains to plant next season's crop.

The onion never lasts that long because we eat it all!

CHILI (DRY)

There will come a time in summer where your chili plants are laden with fruit. This is a good time to pull a few off and place them on the kitchen shelves to dry out. Don't remove any of the seeds or trip the stem, just allow them to dry out completely prior to storing in glass jars. Crushing a whole dried chili with a mortar and pestle and adding that to any meal will give it a lovely kick.

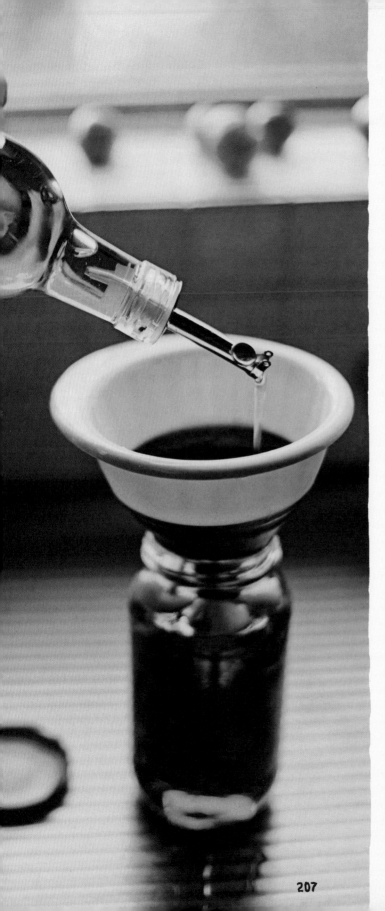

CHILI IN OIL

In our climate we can't grow chili in winter. It's just not a plant that evolved to endure our cold winters. But nothing warms the heart like a hot chili-centric meal in the guts of winter. So a yearly tradition of mine is to store the leftover chilies from the warm season in a bath of olive oil for use over the winter. The beauty of storing them this way is that not only do you preserve the chili, but also you make super hot, chili-infused oil that can be used in place of fresh chili in the cold months.

WHAT YOU NEED:

As many chilies as you want to
    store. Mixed variety is fine.
Empty, sanitized, sealable jars.
Extra-virgin olive oil

HOW TO:

Wash you chilies and drain well until completely dry.

Cut a slit down each chili from top to bottom.

Place in sanitized jars and cover with olive oil.

Wash your hands well after handling the chilies, and DEFINTELY prior to going to the toilet.

PESTO OF BASIL

I BET MOST EVERYONE HAS EATEN THIS PESTO BEFORE, AND SOME HAVE PROBABLY BOUGHT THAT SALTY VERSION YOU CAN BUY IN A JAR, BUT NOTHING BEATS MAKING YOUR OWN!

BASIL SITS COMFORTABLY NEXT TO TOMATOES AS MY FAVORITE SUMMER PLANT. WE PLANT OUT A HUGE CROP OF IT, WITH ENOUGH TO KEEP OUR PLATES HAPPY ALL SUMMER, AND ALSO PLENTY LEFT OVER FOR US TO MAKE PESTO AND TO DRY SOME FOR THE COOLER MONTHS WHEN BASIL (RIGHTLY) REFUSES TO GROW! IF YOU'RE A BASIL LOVER LIKE I AM AND YOU HAVE A HERB GARDEN, I RECOMMEND A FEW STAGGERED PLANTINGS OVER THE WARM MONTHS TO MAKE THE MOST OF THE GROWING SEASON AND AVOID A GLUT.

PART OF THE WLL SYSTEM, IS LEARNING HOW TO CAPTURE SUMMER AND STORE IT FOR THOSE MONTHS IN WINTER WHEN THINGS IN THE PATCH ARE ON THE LIGHT SIDE. WE HAVE PESTO MAKING SESSIONS WHERE WE LOOK LIKE DRUG LORDS, STUFFING ZIPLOC BAGS FULL OF RICH PESTO TO FREEZE. THANKS TO THESE SUMMERTIME EFFORTS, ALL WINTER LONG WE CAN COOK UP PESTO PASTA ON A WHIM WHEN THERE IS NO FRESH BASIL AVAILABLE.

WE MAKE A VARIETY OF PESTOS AND EACH WORKS BEST WITH PARTICULAR INGREDIENTS: FOR EXAMPLE BASIL PESTO WORKS WELL WITH PRAWNS, AND ROCKET AND WILD NETTLE WORK SUPERBLY WITH BROCCOLI. THE KEY TO GOOD TASTING PESTO IS QUALITY INGREDIENTS. STORE-BOUGHT, PRE-GRATED PARMESAN CHEESE ISN'T GOING TO MAKE A SNAZZY PESTO, SO BUY A BLOCK OF EITHER ROMANO OR PARMIGIANINO AND GRATE IT YOURSELF.

WHAT YOU NEED:

1 x handful, fresh basil

1/3 cup (50 g) cashews

1/3 cup (50 g) pine nuts

1.33 cups (150 g) Parmesan, grated

1/3 cup olive oil

Salt

Pepper

HOW TO:

Wash the basil and drain.

In a food processor whiz the nuts. Scrape and remove from the processor.

Whiz the basil into a fine pulp, then return the processed nuts and add the cheese.

Keep blending. As this is all being processed, drizzle in the oil until you get a lovely, thick yet smooth consistency.

Season to taste.

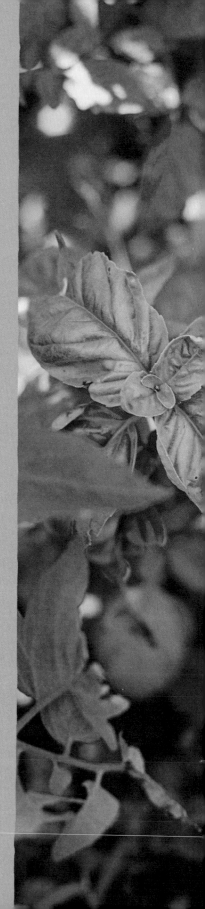

PESTO OF ROCKET

EACH WINTER WE PLANT SPREADING ROCKET, AND IT'S CALLED THAT FOR A VERY SENSIBLE REASON—IT GROWS LIKE WILDFIRE. IT WILL HAPPILY GROW IN THE COLD OF WINTER, AND WILL EVEN SURVIVE THE ODD FROST. IT'S A GREAT PEPPERY ADDITION TO A SALAD, BUT IT'S ALSO USEFUL IN A LESS OBVIOUS WAY, AS A PESTO. NORMALLY BY SPRING OUR BED OF ROCKET IS OUT OF CONTROL AND NO MATTER HOW MUCH WE CONSUME, THERE IS ALWAYS PLENTY LEFT. MAKING PESTO BEGAN AS A NECESSITY, TO TRY TO USE IT ALL BEFORE IT ROTS.

PESTO CAN BE MADE IN BATCHES AND TAGGED AND BAGGED FOR THE FREEZER LIKE FBI EVIDENCE. THIS PESTO CAN BE USED AS PASTA DRESSING OR AS DIP; EITHER WAY YOU'LL NEVER THINK OF ROCKET AS JUST A SALAD LEAF AGAIN.

WHAT YOU NEED:

2 x large handfuls fresh rocket
3/4 cup dried sunflower seeds
2 x fresh chili, diced (optional)
3.5 oz (100 g) feta cheese
3 tbsp Philadelphia cream cheese
1/4 cup olive oil
Salt
Pepper

HOW TO:

Wash the freshly picked rocket and pat dry.

Mash up the sunflower seeds in a food processer until relatively smooth and remove into a bowl.

Puree the rocket in the food processor. Mash it really well before adding the feta and grated Parmesan cheese.

Return the mashed sunflower seeds to the processor along with the Philadelphia and fresh chili. Keep whizzing.

While mixing, gradually add the olive oil to make a thick paste. Add more olive oil as required.

Season to taste.

Store in freezer bags or a sealed plastic tube for freezer storage.

PESTO OF PARSLEY

THERE SEEMS TO BE SOME DEBATE ABOUT WHETHER FLAT LEAF PARSLEY IS BETTER THAN CURLY. SERIOUSLY? IT'S BLOODY PARSLEY—STOP BEING SO DAMN PRECIOUS! IT TASTES GREAT, IT'S GOOD FOR YOU, WHY WOULD YOU NOT WANT TO GROW IT? EITHER VARIETY. WHEN YOU HAVE PLENTY GROWING, MAKE A FEW BATCHES OF THIS PESTO. EAT SOME FRESH WITH PASTA, USE AS A DIP, OR AS A SPREAD WITH MEAT. IT'S PRETTY VERSATILE.

WHAT YOU NEED:

2 x bunches parsley
1 cup toasted pine nuts
1 cup parmesan/pecorino, grated
3.25 oz (100 g) feta
1 x lemon rind
1 x lemon juice
1/2 cup olive oil
Salt
Pepper

HOW TO:

Panfry the pine nuts in a little bit of olive oil for a few minutes until they're almost golden brown. Remove from heat.

Whiz the parsley in a food processor and remove.

Process the toasted pines.

Return the parsley to the machine. Crumble in the feta, add the Parmesan, the rind of lemon, and the lemon juice. Process.

As the machine is spinning, pour in the olive oil gradually until the consistency is just right, and season to taste.

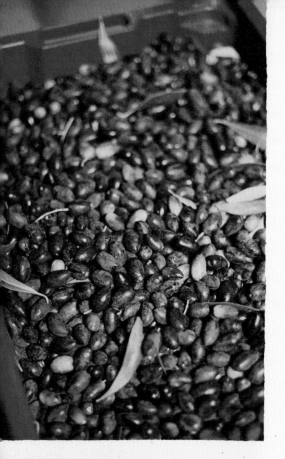

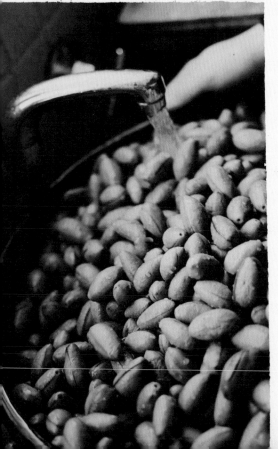

PICKLING OLIVES

There are two basic ways I process our handpicked olives, a dry way and a wet way. Both require salt. You also need some pretty high tech equipment: a large plastic bucket and a cane basket. Both methods described below use about 4.5 lb (2 kg) of olives.

THE WET WAY

First, you need to cut a slit on both sides of the olives lengthways. If you want you can crush the olives with the bottom of a beer bottle (preferably empty, that is unless you want to offer that beer to an enemy immediately after the olive crushing job is done).

By opening the skin the salt is able to penetrate the flesh and remove the bitterness more effectively. Drop them in the bucket.

If you want to be super fancy, you can buy a pitting machine. I haven't reached that level of sophistication yet.

So now you've had a session of olive slitting or crushing and you have some olives in a bucket. Go fill that bucket with cold water and a handful of salt (about a tbsp).

For the next two weeks or longer, change the water every few days until that fresh-olive bitterness is removed. This takes a few seasons to perfect.

Remove the olives. Wash and rinse well under running water.

Store in sanitized jars in a saline solution of 1/3 cup (100 g) salt per quart (1 liter) of water.

THE DRY WAY

I use this method for smaller, black olives like Manzanillo or kalamata.

Place the olives in the basket. Cover them with dry salt for a few weeks.

After two weeks, taste an olive to check for bitterness.

Store in sanitized jars and fill with olive oil.

Optional (for both methods): Add garlic, peppercorns, and/or chili to the jars.

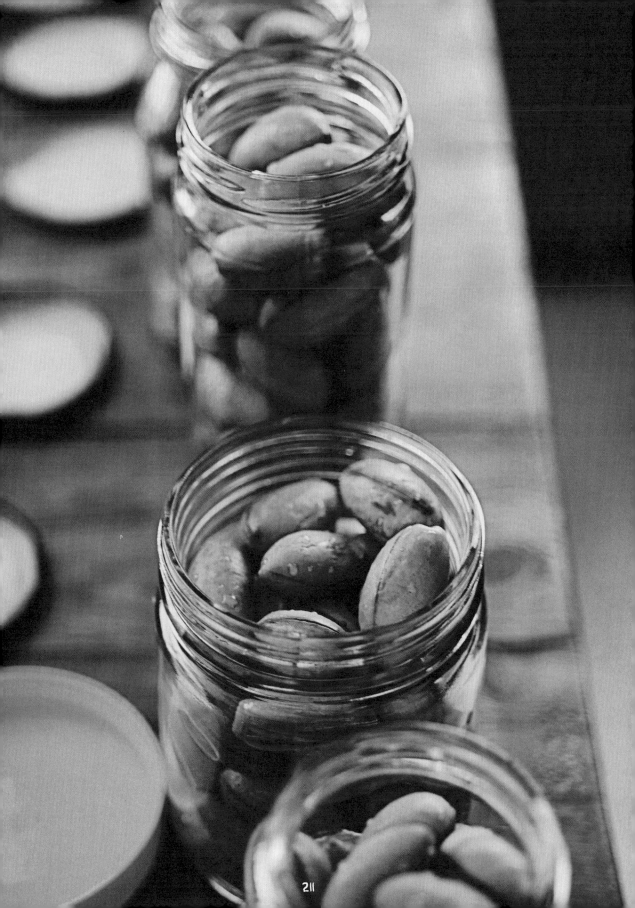

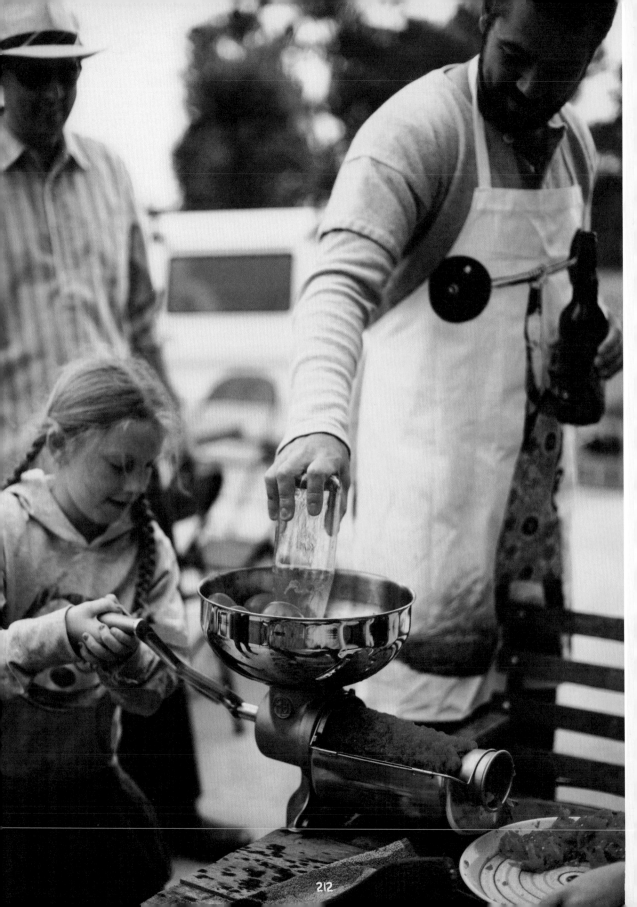

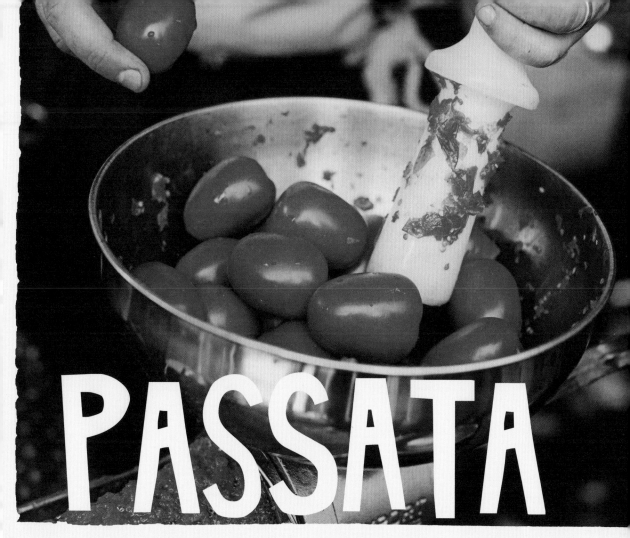

PASSATA

TOMATO PASSATA IS SUCH AN INTEGRAL PART OF THE WLL SYSTEM. IT'S A TRADITION WE PICKED UP FROM ITALIAN-AUSTRALIAN FAMILIES THAT MAKE "PASSATA DAY" A FAMILY FESTIVAL EACH HARVEST SEASON, USUALLY IN AUTUMN. IT'S A GREAT DAY TO CELEBRATE EVERYTHING THAT THE RIPE TOMATO REPRESENTS, VIBRANT COLOR, SUMMER FLAVOR, AND THE SYMBOL OF A GOOD HARVEST. PASSATA IS BEST STORED IN BEER BOTTLES OR HOME BREWING BOTTLES BUT NO MATTER WHAT, THEY MUST BE GLASS AND YOU MUST CAP THE LIDS FIRMLY. UNLIKE ROASTED PASSATA, THE BOILED METHOD DOES REQUIRE A FRUIT CRUSHING MACHINE THAT CAN EITHER BE RENTED OR PURCHASED AT MOST ITALIAN FOOD SPECIALTY SHOPS OR ONLINE. WE USE A HAND CRANK MACHINE, WHICH WORKS EFFICIENTLY AND IS FUN FOR EVERYONE TO HAVE A GO WITH.

TO MAKE THE DAY WORTHWHILE, WE START WITH AT LEAST 100 LB (50 KG) OF FRESH TOMATOES. THIS IS A CHALLENGE TO GROW IN A SMALL YARD SO WE OFTEN USE A MIXTURE OF OUR PRODUCE AND LOCALLY GROWN COMMERCIAL VARIETIES. THIS WILL MAKE ENOUGH PASSATA FOR A FAMILY OF FOUR FOR AN ENTIRE YEAR.

THIS METHOD ALSO PRODUCES A MORE RUNNY CONSISTENCY, BUT DOES REDUCE ON HEAT VERY WELL.

ROASTING TOMATO TO MAKE PASSATA WAS MY FIRST APPROACH. WHEN I'D HAVE A FEW KILOS MORE THAN I NEEDED I'D ROAST THEM AND MAKE A QUICK SAUCE THAT WOULD GET USED DURING THE WEEK. ROASTING THE TOMATOES INSTEAD OF BOILING THEM BRINGS OUT THE SWEETNESS OF THE FRUIT, ESPECIALLY IF YOU HAVE PLENTY OF BEAUTIFUL LITTLE CHERRY TOMATOES. IT'S A VERY SIMPLE PROCESS AND ONCE YOU'VE MADE IT YOU'LL BE SURE TO RETURN TO IT AS AN OLD FAVORITE.

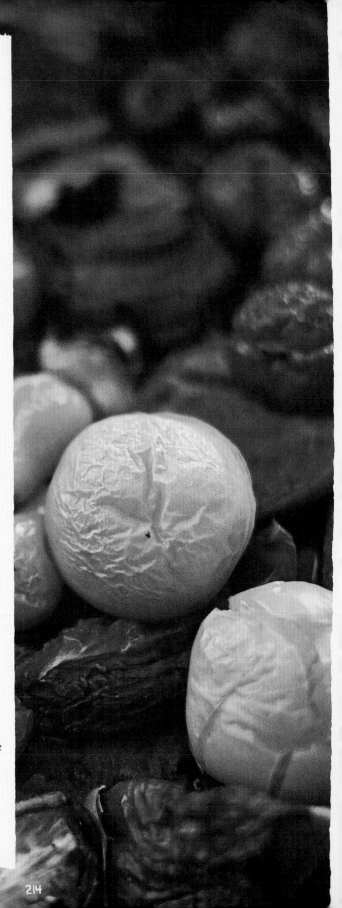

ROASTED TOMATO PASSATA

5–10 lb (2-4 kg) fresh, mixed tomato
1 large bunch fresh basil
10 x garlic cloves
Olive oil
Salt
Cracked pepper

HOW TO:

Preheat the oven to 400 F (200 C).

Roughly slice the tomatoes and lay out on a large roasting tray (you may need a few).

Peel the garlic, but leave whole. Add to the roasting tray.

Roughly chop half the basil and add it to the tray.

Generously drizzle the tomato with olive oil, crack over some salt and pepper, and roast for 45 minutes or until a little charring starts to occur.

Remove from the oven and allow too cool.

Using a fine, steel sieve and a large cooking spoon, push the roasted tomatoes through the colander into a large bowl.

When complete, finely chop up the remaining basil and stir through the sauce.

Transfer into containers and refrigerate.

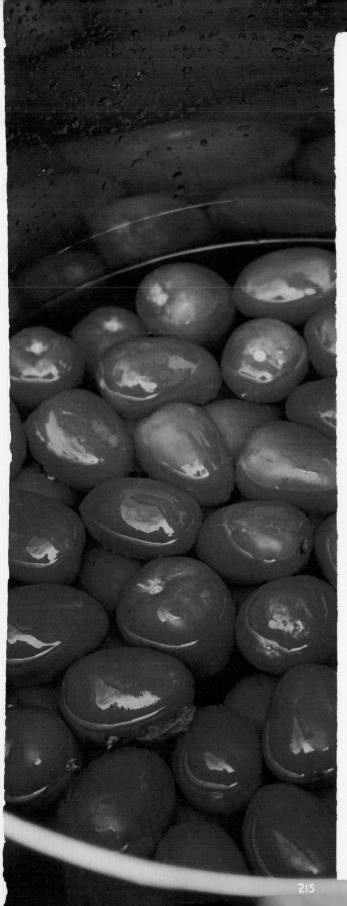

BOILED TOMATO PASSATA

WHAT YOU NEED:

Over 100 lb (50 kg) fresh tomato
Fresh basil

HOW TO:

Boil tomatoes in around 20 lb (10 kg)
batches for at least 5 minutes to soften them.

Crush them in the fruit crusher, collecting the
sauce in large pots. Run the pulped tomatoes
through at least twice.

Pour into sterilized beer bottles, leaving a few
inches unfilled at the top. Place a basil leaf in
each bottle prior to capping it.

Once all the bottles are filled and tightly capped,
gently stack them in 40 gallon drums set up on a
brick frame, with space between the bricks,
 about four bricks high. Use old towels or cardboard between the bottles to avoid breakages.
Make sure the drum is secure in place.

Fill the drum with cold water, then start a good
wood fire underneath and keep it going for 5
hours, or until the water has been at its boiling
point for an hour or so.

Allow the water to cool overnight and remove
the bottles the following day. Be warned,
it is inevitable that some bottles will break
with the heating process, so be careful when
removing them.

Store the bottles in a dark larder.

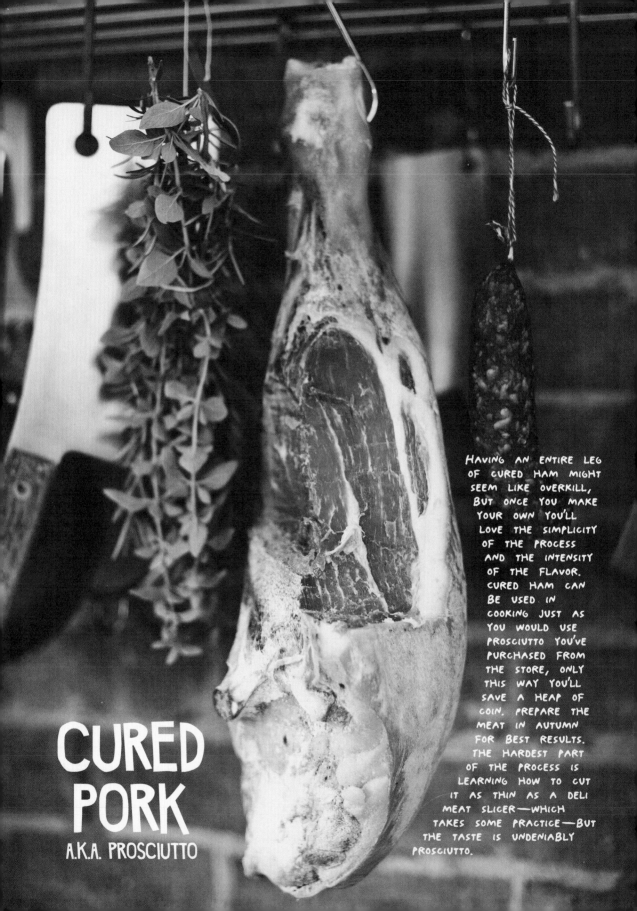

CURED PORK
A.K.A. PROSCIUTTO

HAVING AN ENTIRE LEG OF CURED HAM MIGHT SEEM LIKE OVERKILL, BUT ONCE YOU MAKE YOUR OWN YOU'LL LOVE THE SIMPLICITY OF THE PROCESS AND THE INTENSITY OF THE FLAVOR. CURED HAM CAN BE USED IN COOKING JUST AS YOU WOULD USE PROSCIUTTO YOU'VE PURCHASED FROM THE STORE, ONLY THIS WAY YOU'LL SAVE A HEAP OF COIN. PREPARE THE MEAT IN AUTUMN FOR BEST RESULTS. THE HARDEST PART OF THE PROCESS IS LEARNING HOW TO CUT IT AS THIN AS A DELI MEAT SLICER—WHICH TAKES SOME PRACTICE—BUT THE TASTE IS UNDENIABLY PROSCIUTTO.

WHAT YOU NEED:

17.5 lb (8 kg) leg of pork
30–40 lb (15–20 kg) cooking salt
Large plastic tub with lid
Wooden hanging cage, sealed, with fly screen
Butcher's hook
New rubber gloves
Patience

HOW TO: (PREPARE IN AUTUMN)

Wearing gloves, rub salt over the entire leg; give it a good rub in.

Place the leg in the large plastic tub and cover the whole thing in salt. Cover the tub. The general rule is top let it cure one day per kilo (roughly half a day per pound) but I've left it in the salt for over 25 days with the same result.

At the end of the salting period, remove the leg from the tub and brush off the salt.

In your tailor-made hanging cage, hang the leg by the butchers hook around the knuckle of the foot.

Make sure the cage is totally sealed and no insects can get in.

Store in a cellar or shed where the temperature at humidity remains fairly constant.

Leave the leg to hang for 9-12 months, the longer you leave it cure the more complex the flavor that will develop.

Mold will form on the outside of the leg during the curing phase. Don't dispose of your meat, it's totally normal. Yes, it's a bit manky, but as long as you don't get large green mold forming you should be okay. There will be little white and black bits of mold on the skin, and all of this will be cut off and removed when you cut the leg open to get to the good stuff.

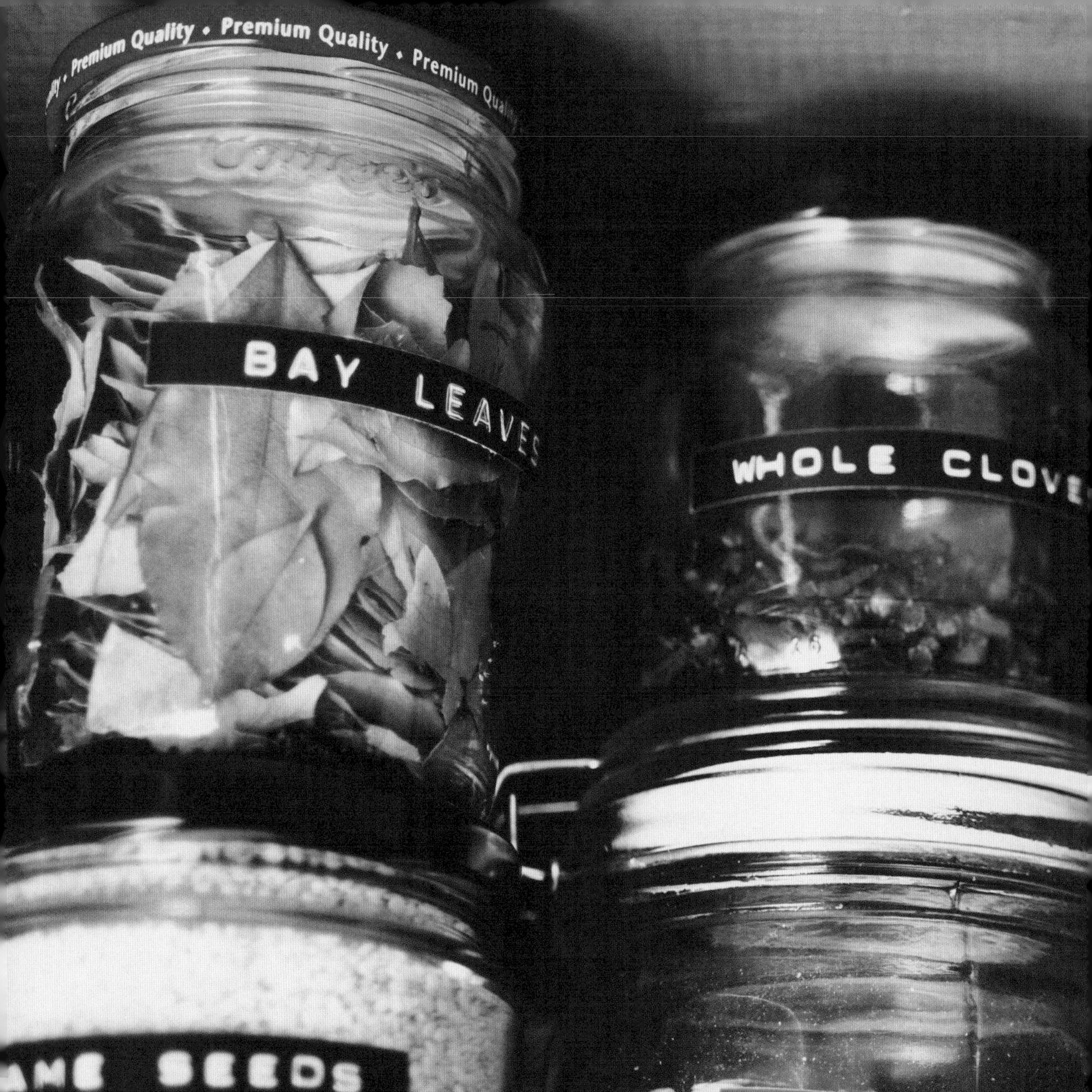

BAY LEAVES

WHOLE CLOVE

AME SEEDS

SUNFLOWER

I LOVE USING FRESH HERBS, BUT FOR SOME HERBS THEY WORK JUST AS WELL DRIED.
I'LL OFTEN PICK SOME THYME OR ROSEMARY AND HANG IT FOR A FEW WEEKS TO DRY,
THEN I'LL CRUNCH THE LEAVES OFF AND USED THEM WHEN ROASTING CHICKEN AND SPUDS.
CORIANDER AND GARLIC ARE TWO OTHER PLANTS THAT I LIKE TO LET GO TO SEED, THEN PICK
THE SEEDS AND USE THEM IN THE KITCHEN, WHILE SOME OTHER HERBS I'LL ONLY USE FRESH.

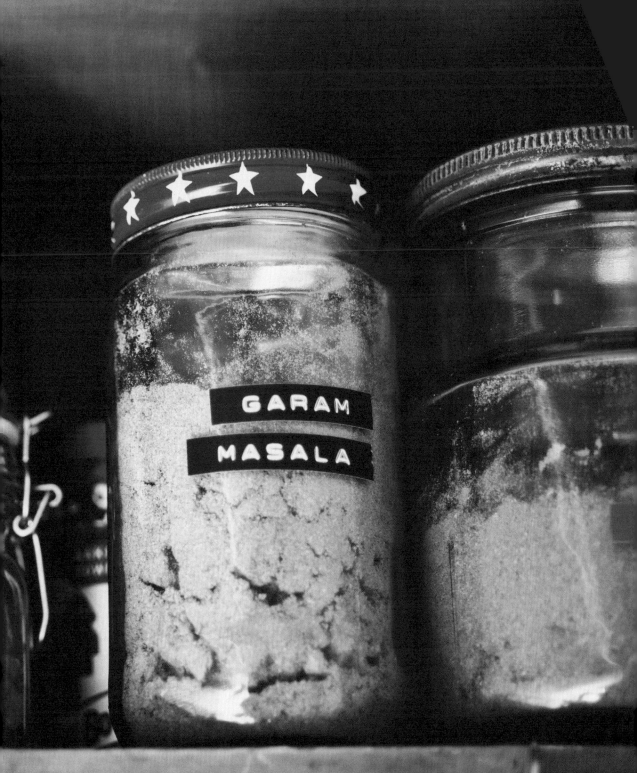

GARAM
MASALA

ODD LITTLE FELLA,
AREN'T I?

BOYSENBERRY + RASPBERRY JAM

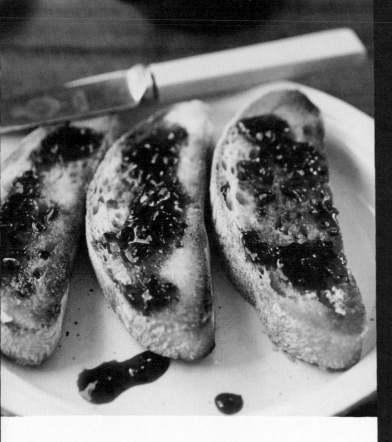

THIS IS ONE OF THE HARDEST JAMS TO MAKE. IT'S NOT THE COOKING PROCESS ITSELF THAT'S DIFFICULT, BUT REFRAINING FROM DEVOURING THE BERRIES WHEN YOU'RE PICKING THEM OFF THE VINE. THE "ONE FOR THE BUCKET ONE FOR ME" APPROACH TO HARVESTING CAN BE RATHER DETRIMENTAL IN REGARDS TO EFFICIENCY.

I LOVE MAKING JAMS IN SUMMER, KNOWING THAT MY TOASTED BREAD WILL BE IN GOOD COMPANY ON THE COLD MORNINGS OF WINTER, MY PANCAKES WILL BE IMPROVED, AND SCONES WILL GET THE SWEETNESS THEY DESERVE. THE COOKING PROCESS IS SIMPLE, BUT THERE ARE A FEW THINGS THAT YOU SHOULD PAY ATTENTION TO. FIRSTLY, MAKE SURE YOUR JARS ARE REALLY STERILIZED. SOME DISHWASHING MACHINES HAVE A STERILIZING SETTING. IF NOT, YOU CAN DIP YOUR JARS IN BOILING WATER FOR A FEW MINUTES AND REMOVE WITH TONGS. THE SECOND THING TO REMEMBER IS CONSISTENCY OF YOUR JAM. YOU WANT TO GET THE THICKNESS RIGHT AND NOT MAKE A SUPER RUNNY JAM; THERE IS A LITTLE TRICK TO THIS AND IT'S ACHIEVED BY COOKING THE FRUIT TO RELEASE THE NATURAL PECTIN, WHICH GIVES IT THAT JELLY-LIKE CONSISTENCY. THEY TRICK IS NOT COOKING THE JAM TOO LONG AS TO REDUCE THE PECTIN'S EFFECTIVENESS. THE BEST WAY TO CHECK FOR THICKNESS IS AFTER SIMMERING FOR THE REQUIRED TIME, TAKE A SPOONFUL AND PLACE IT ON A SMALL PLATE. THEN POP IT IN THE FREEZER FOR FIVE MINUTES. IF, WHEN COOLED, THE JAM IS THICK ON THE PLATE AND STICKS TOGETHER TO YOUR PREFERENCE, THEN IT'S READY TO BOTTLE.

WHAT YOU NEED:

Roughly 1 lb (500 g) boysenberry

Roughly 1 lb (500 g) raspberry

A little over 2 lb (1 kg) sugar

1 x lemon juice

1 x quill cinnamon

HOW TO:

Rinse you fruit and strain dry.

In a large pot, add the fruit, sugar, cinnamon, and lemon juice.

Bring to a boil and simmer for 40 minutes.

Remove cinnamon stick.

When you have your desired consistency bottle in sterilized jars.

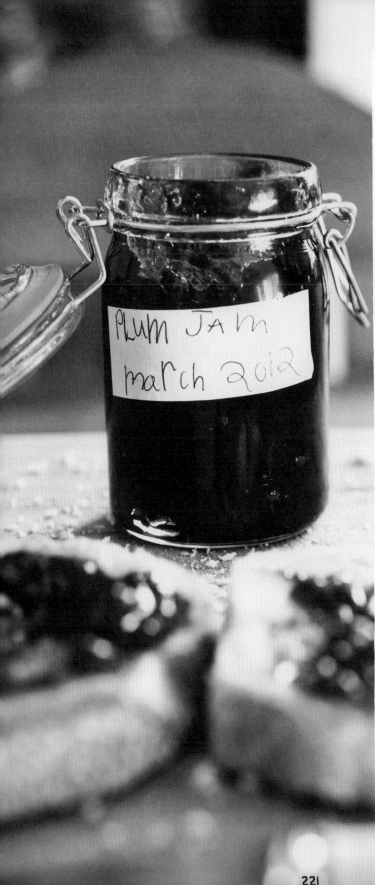

BLOOD PLUM JAM

BLOOD PLUMS ARE A DELICIOUS TREAT STRAIGHT OFF THE BRANCH, BUT WHEN YOU HAVE A FEW POUNDS TO SPARE, MAKING A JAM IS AN EXCELLENT WAY TO BOOST YOUR STORES FOR WINTER. I LOVE THIS JAM PRESENTED SIMPLY ON FRESH BAKED BREAD, BUT IT CAN GO INTO SMOOTHIES, ON TOP OF PANCAKES, AND WITH ICE CREAM.

IF YOU CAN'T GET BLOOD PLUMS SPECIFICALLY, USE WHATEVER PLUMP PLUMS YOU CAN PROCURE.

WHAT YOU NEED:

5 lb (2 kg) blood plums
3 1/4 lb (1.5 kg) raw sugar
1 x quill cinnamon

HOW TO:

Rinse the plums under water and then slice them with a small knife and remove the pits.

Pop into a large pot with the sugar and the cinnamon quill and bring to a boil.

Simmer on a low heat for 40 minutes until a thick, rich sauce consistency is achieved.

Store in sterilized jars.

SEMI-DRIED TOMATOES

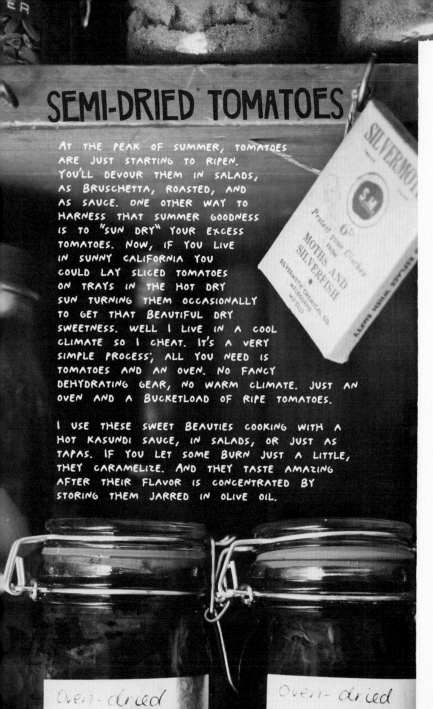

At the peak of summer, tomatoes are just starting to ripen. You'll devour them in salads, as bruschetta, roasted, and as sauce. One other way to harness that summer goodness is to "sun dry" your excess tomatoes. Now, if you live in sunny California you could lay sliced tomatoes on trays in the hot dry sun turning them occasionally to get that beautiful dry sweetness. Well I live in a cool climate so I cheat. It's a very simple process; all you need is tomatoes and an oven. No fancy dehydrating gear, no warm climate. Just an oven and a bucketload of ripe tomatoes.

I use these sweet beauties cooking with a hot kasundi sauce, in salads, or just as tapas. If you let some burn just a little, they caramelize. And they taste amazing after their flavor is concentrated by storing them jarred in olive oil.

Oven-dried tomatoes march 12

Oven-dried tomatoes Mar 1a

WHAT YOU NEED:

Ripe tomatoes
Olive oil

HOW TO:

Slice the tomatoes lengthwise into 4–6 slices (depending on the size of the tomatoes).

Don't worry about the seeds, if some fall out, no matter.

Take the tray grills out from the oven and preheat the oven to the lowest setting. For my oven it's 150 F (60 C), convection.

Here's the trick. Jam a pencil in the door so the oven isn't sealed

Lay the sliced tomatoes directly on the wire racks and return to the low-heat, semi-opened oven and roast until they shrivel up and some even char a little. This should only take around and hour, but check on them regularly.

Allow to cool.

Transfer the tomatoes into sterilized jars and fill with olive oil ensuring all tomatoes are covered. Allow oil to sink and fill into all the cracks between the tomatoes and top up if necessary as any tomatoes exposed may spoil.

CHILI-PICKLED WILD MUSHROOMS

PRESERVING MUSHROOMS HAS ALWAYS MEANT DRYING FOR ME; THAT IS UNTIL I WAS HANDED A JAR OF PICKLED MUSHROOMS BY A FORAGING FRIEND. THEY'RE A SPECIAL TREAT AS ANTIPASTI, AND CAN ALSO BE USED IN DISHES. SOME FOLKS MAY NOT LIKE THE TEXTURE OR THE PEPPERY TANG, BUT I LOVE BOTH. IF YOU'RE A KEEN MUSHROOM HUNTER YOU CAN USE ALL THE TINY MUSHROOMS YOU FIND AND KEEP THEM WHOLE OR JUST SLICED IN HALF. IF NOT, JUST SLICE UP LARGER MUSHROOMS.

WHAT YOU NEED:

5 cups sliced mushrooms
1 x large onion, chopped
5 x cloves garlic
1 x jalapeño pepper, sliced (seeds in)
1 cup vinegar
Fresh bay leaf
1 tbsp black peppercorns
1 tbsp yellow mustard seed
Salt

HOW TO:

Boil the sliced mushrooms for 10 minutes, drain, and lay out to dry on a paper towel.

When dry, transfer to sterilized jars along with the sliced onion, whole garlic cloves, and jalapeño.

In a saucepan bring the vinegar to a boil with the mustard seeds, peppercorns, and bay leaf.

Pour the hot, liquid mix over the mushrooms in the jar and leave sealed for a few weeks until the flavors work their way into the mushrooms.

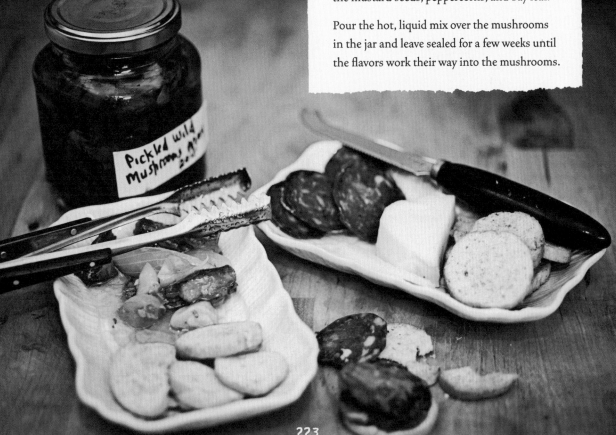

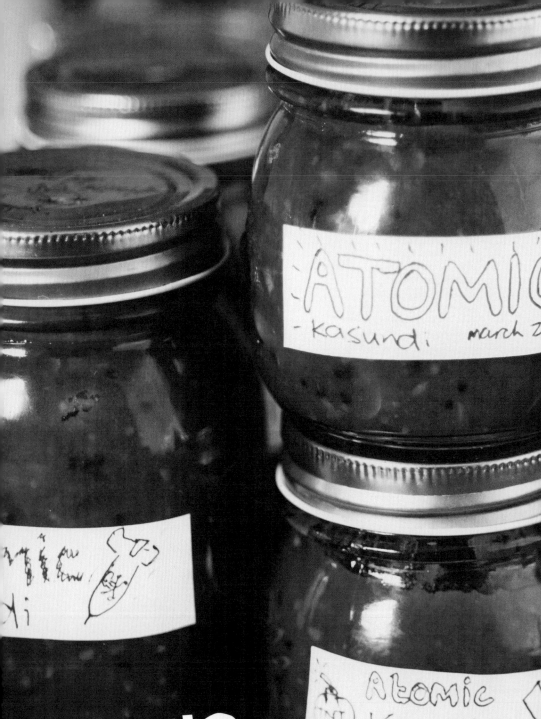

ATOMIC
KASUNDI

I'M PRETTY SURE THAT THE TERM KASUNDI IS JUST BENGALI FOR "SAUCE" OR SOMETHING ALONG THOSE LINES SO I'M PROBABLY MAKING A LOT OF DIFFERENT TYPES OF KASUNDI WITH THE AMOUNT OF TOMATO BASED CHUTNEY I MAKE AT THE END OF EACH SUMMER. THIS VERSION IS SOMETHING THAT CAUGHT MY TASTE BUDS WHEN I BOUGHT A JAR OF IT OFF A LOVELY LITTLE INDIAN FAMILY AT A SCHOOL FETE, AND IT BLEW MY SOCKS OFF! GREAT HEAT FROM PLENTY OF CHILI AND THE SWEET GINGER AND TOMATO COMBO HAD ME IN LOVE STRAIGHT AWAY. I KNEW I SHOULD HAVE BOUGHT MORE THAN JUST ONE JAR. I HAD THAT JAR OF KASUNDI ON EVERYTHING; TOASTED FOCCACIA, BURGERS, ROAST MEAT, BBQ CHICKEN, AND ESPECIALLY LOVED IT SERVED ON A SLICE OF CRUMBLY AGED CHEDDAR. SO I HAD TO FIGURE OUT HOW TO MAKE MY OWN. NOW, I'M NOT A CHILI EATING CHAMPION, BUT I DO LOVE HEAT. SO, IF YOU'RE NOT A FAN OF TOO MUCH HEAT THEN YOU CAN TONE IT DOWN WITH LESS CHILI OR USE A LESS VOLATILE TYPE OF CHILI. I'VE BEEN GROWING A LITTLE ATOMIC CHILI (NOT ACTUAL NAME) THAT I BOUGHT A FEW YEARS AGO AND JUST COLLECT THE SEED EACH YEAR. DON'T BE FOOLED BY CHILI, SOMETIMES THE SMALLER THEY GET THE HOTTER THEY ARE. I MAKE THIS KASUNDI WHEN I HAVE A FEW KILOS OF FRESH TOMATOES ALL RIPE AT THE SAME TIME. THE RECIPE BELOW ISN'T FOR THE FAINT OF HEART, BUT IT'S EASY TO ADJUST BY REGULATING THE AMOUNT OF CHILI YOU ADD.

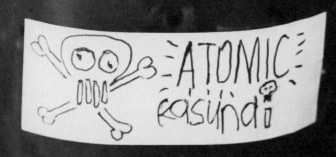

WHAT YOU NEED:

- 6.5 lb (3 kg) ripe tomatoes, skins removed
- 20 x cloves garlic, diced
- 7 x hot chilies, diced (seeds in)
- 3 cups malt vinegar
- 2.5 cups sugar
- 10 oz (300 g) ginger, grated
- 6 tbsp mixed mustard seeds
- 6 tbsp cumin
- 3 tbsp turmeric
- 1 tbsp chili powder
- 3 tbsp sunflower oil

HOW TO:

Cut an X at one end of the tomatoes—preferably the end withou the vine attachment.

Pop them in boiling water for a minute then remove into a colander to cool.

Peel off the skins and dice.

In a large pot add the spices to the sunflower oil and heat for a few minutes.

Add the diced tomato, ginger, garlic, and chili and mix well.

Add the sugar and malt vinegar and simmer for 45 minutes.

Store in sterilized jars and leave for a few weeks to brew the flavors.

DILL PICKLED CUCUMBERS

THERE ARE ALL SORTS OF CUCUMBERS YOU CAN GROW. I TENDED TO STICK WITH THE LEBANESE VARIETY ONLY BECAUSE IT'S WHAT I GREW UP WITH. THAT IS UNTIL SOMEONE SHARED SOME SEEDS TO GROW DILL-PICKLING CUCUMBERS WITH ME. THEY WERE PROLIFIC! I DIDN'T NEED TO DO MUCH FOR THEM—JUST POPPED THEM IN THE GROUND AND WATERED THEM. THEY SEEM TO FLOWER ALL SUMMER (PRETTY PLANT AND FLOWERS TOO) AND THE AMOUNT OF FRUIT OFF ONE PLANT IS ASTONISHING! INTRIGUED BY THE "FACT" THAT THEY WERE DILL-PICKLE VARIETY, I DECIDED TO ATTEMPT TO PICKLE SOME AND WAS DELIGHTED WHEN I OPENED THE FIRST JAR AFTER IMPATIENTLY WAITING THE NORMAL FEW WEEKS TO ALLOW THE VINEGAR TO WORK IT'S MAGIC. THESE TURNED OUT BETTER THAN STORE-BOUGHT. THEY WORK THEIR BEST ON A HAMBURGER—THAT'S A NO BRAINER. BUT THEY ALSO WORK WELL ON TOASTED FOCACCIA WITH GOOD, HONEY-ROASTED HAM OR BASICALLY ANY MEAT AND CHEESE. LETS FACE IT, IF YOU LIKE GHERKIN YOU'LL EAT THEM WITH ALMOST ANYTHING. OKAY, NOT YOGURT. WHATEVER.

WHAT YOU NEED:

Cucumbers (all sizes and shapes, but see if you can get the variety best suited to pickling)

2 x onion, chopped

8 x cloves garlic

2 x large fresh chilli

1 quart (1 liter) white vinegar

2–3 cups (500–700 ml) apple cider vinegar

1 cup sugar

2 tbsp dried dill

1.5 tbsp black mustard seed

1.5 tbsp yellow mustard seed

1 tbsp black peppercorn

1/2 tbsp dried fennel seed

1/2 tbsp turmeric

Cooking salt

HOW TO:

Slice the cucumbers lengthwise into thin pieces. Do the same with the onions. Place in a large mixing bowl and sprinkle with cooking salt and toss. If you have small whole cucumbers (3–4 inches long), pop them in whole.

Cover and leave for two hours.

Drain the liquid that has gathered from the bowl.

Place all the cucumbers into sterilized jars with the dill.

Pop all the other ingredients in a pot and bring to a boil.

Stir the mix well and then while hot, pour over the cucumbers in the jars and seal the lids tightly. Flip the jars upside down to ensure they don't leak.

Store for a minimum of 2 weeks before opening.

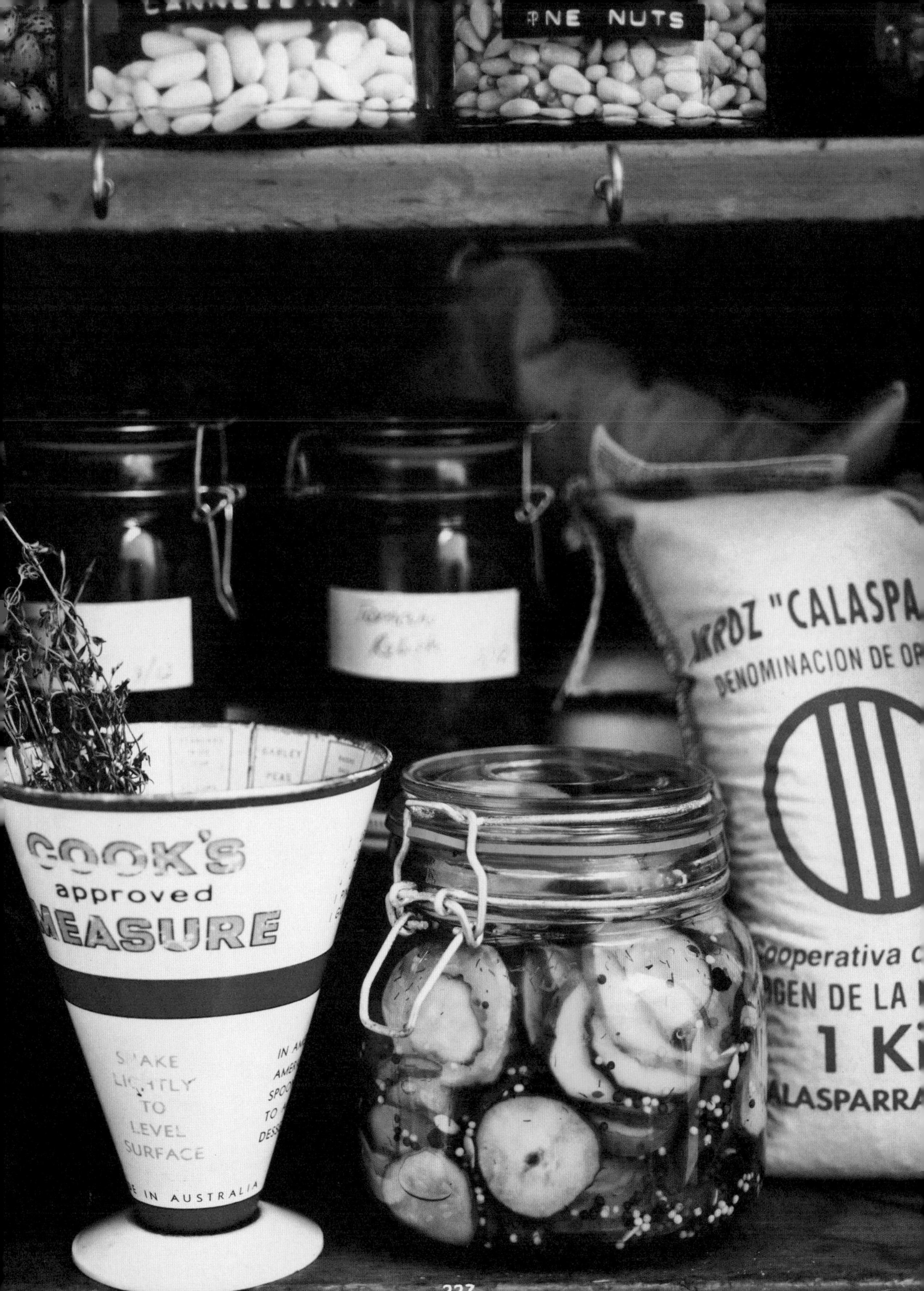
NUTS
COOK'S
approved
MEASURE
LIGHTLY
TO
LEVEL
SURFACE
IN AUSTRALIA
"CALASPA
DENOMINACION DE O
Cooperativa
GEN DE LA
1 Ki
ALASPARRA

SOME

BASICS

Here are very basic versions of things I like to make. Yes I eat a lot of pasta and bread.

PASTA: EGG NOODLES

Mix together 1 egg per 1 cup (100 g) of 00 flour. I normally make a minimum of 500 g, which means I use 5 eggs.

Knead well for at least 10 minutes until tight dough is achieved.

Rest in a flour-dusted bowl, covered, for two hours.

Cut into small sized balls and roll out per your pasta machine's instructions: roll, fold, roll, fold...then finally, cut to desired pasta setting on machine.

Dust immediately with flour.

Cooks in 5 minutes in salted boiling water.

PIZZA BASE

8 cups (800 g) 00 flour (plus some extra for dusting)
3 cups (700 ml) lukewarm water
1/2 oz (14 g) dry yeast
1 tsp caster sugar
Semolina flour

To make the dough for the pizza base, first mix the lukewarm water with the yeast. Add the caster sugar, stir and set aside for at least 5 minutes.

Tip the flour into the bowl of an electric mixer (if using one), or a large bowl if you plan on kneading by hand. Make a fist-sized well in the centre of flour, and then pour the yeast mixture into it. Mix the ingredients until a basic dough forms.

Set the dough onto a flat kneading surface dusted with flour. For 10 minutes, knead the dough by pushing into it with the heel of your hand and then folding the dough in on itself. At about the 8

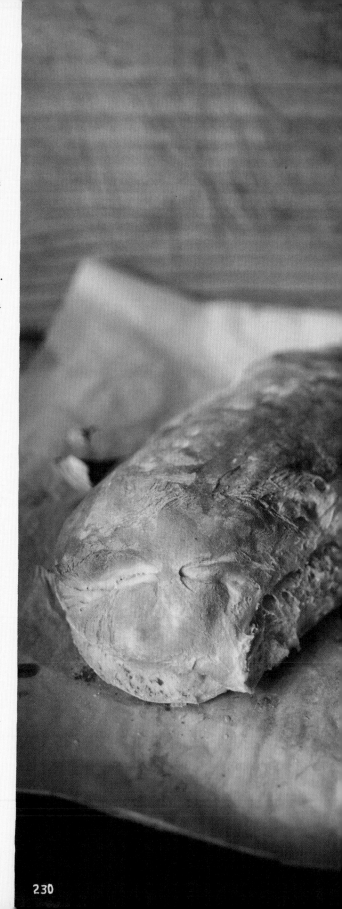

minute mark, the dough should feel smooth and elastic. If necessary, you can add more flour as you knead.

Dust the base of a large bowl with flour, and place the dough inside. Cover the bowl with a tea towel. Let the dough rest and rise for at least 30 minutes, until it has doubled in size.

Separate the dough into 6 to 8 pieces, depending on how large you want each pizza to be. Sprinkle a flat surface with semolina flour, and use a rolling pin to roll each dough ball into a circle shape by pushing from the centre out, all the way around. Aim for an even thickness of about 1/4 in (1/2 cm).

SUPER EASY COUNTRY BREAD

Roughly 1 lb or 5 cups (500 g) plain flour
1 x egg white
3/4 oz or 2.25 tbsp (21 g) yeast, mixed
1.5 cups lukewarm water
A pinch of salt
Olive oil

Mix the yeast in the water and allow it to dissolve for half an hour.

In an electric mixer add the salt and flour. On a slow setting, gradually add the water.

Mix until all ingredients are combined well.

Remove into an oiled bowl, and rest in a warm spot for an hour.

Knead for five minutes, then roll out into two loaves, cover with a towel and let rest for 15 minutes.

Meanwhile, preheat the oven to 375 F (190 C).

Bake the bread for 15 minutes. Remove and brush with the beaten egg white and return to the oven for another 10 minutes.

Allow it to cool for 10 minutes before serving.

BASIC GNOCCHI

6 x washed and peeled potatoes
1 x egg
1 x nutmeg or grated nutmeg
Semolina
Plain flour
Cracked pepper

Peel and boil the potatoes until cooked through. Test with a fork to see if they're soft.

Strain and allow to cool.

Mash them using a potato ricer (best invention ever). If you don't have one then use a steel colander and push the potato through with a soupspoon.

In a mixing bowl, mix the egg, half a grated nutmeg, and a good crack of pepper. Mix well. If you like getting you hands right into it and plenty messy you will love this bit.

On a clean surface, sprinkle a handful of flour and pour the mixture onto it, rolling and adding flour until you have a dough-like consistency.

Once you have achieved this, make long sausage like shapes. Refrain from eating these, as they taste nothing like sausage.

Chop into little gnocchi pieces around an inch long. There are no rules—it's home made, it's supposed to look rustic. If you have plenty of time you can make impressions of a fork on each gnocchi, which when cooked, will help "catch" the sauce.

Lay the pieces of gnocchi on trays on a bed of semolina and rest for a few hours in the fridge to set.

In a large pot bring 2–3 quarts (2–3 liters) of water to boil. Add the gnocchi and stir gently to keep them from sticking.

They will rise to the surface when cooked.

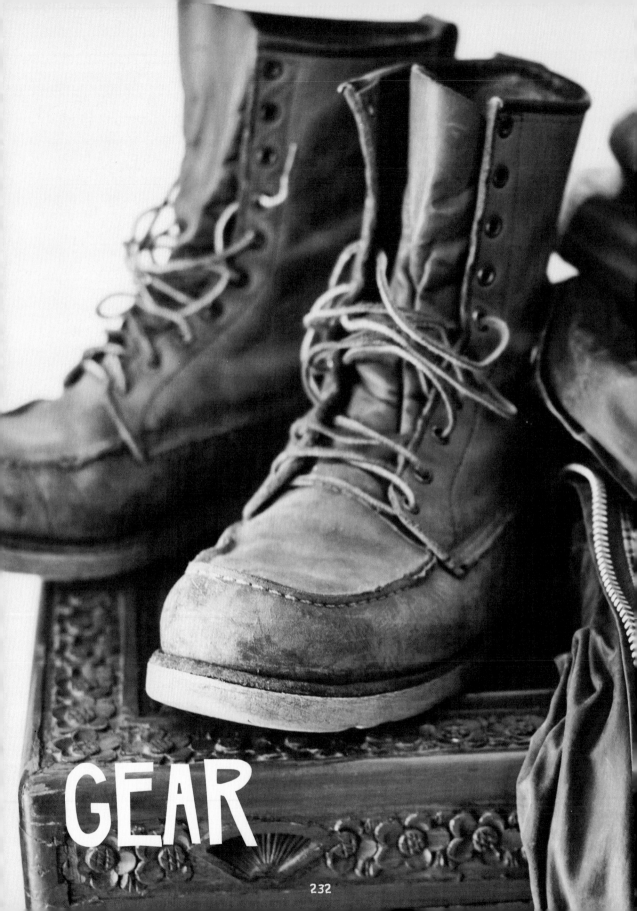

GEAR

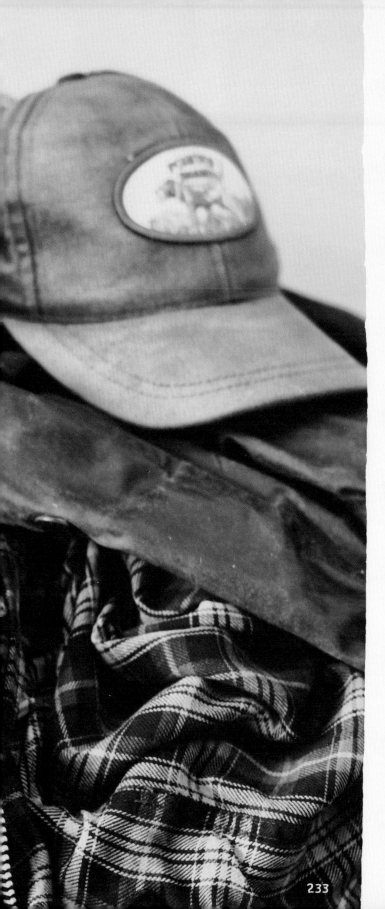

I used to call my brother a gear queer (an affectionate term) for his love of hiking gear, but I think the tables have definitely turned. For the WLL system to work, I've slowly built up an arsenal of gear, things that you may not initially think about but inevitably become a necessity. Your gear acquisition will be dependent on what endeavors you're preparing to undertake; for example, if you're living in a major city in a poky apartment, a large gun safe and full-size rubber waders are probably not necessary. But a range of pots for your rooftop garden might be.

I can't stress this enough: with most things in life you may have to pay extra for quality, after that it's up to you to look after it.

Here's a few things that I could not do without.

KITCHEN KNIVES

WHETHER YOU'RE A CITY DWELLER OR COUNTRY MOUSE, YOU WILL NEED A DECENT KNIFE OR TWO. GET THE GOOD ONES, ASK AROUND FOR ADVICE AND KEEP THEM SHARP. I GO POSTAL TRYING TO USE A BLUNT KNIFE, SERIOUSLY POSTAL... BREATHE IN...BREATHE OUT. I USE THREE MAIN KNIVES ALL VICTORINOX A GENERAL-PURPOSE CHEF'S KNIFE, A BONING KNIFE, AND A BONE-CUTTING KNIFE. BUY THESE NEW AND LOOK AFTER THEM. KEEP THEM SHARP AND THEY WILL REWARD YOU WITH MANY GOOD YEARS IN THE KITCHEN. I HAVE A GUY THAT COMES TO THE HOUSE IN A LITTLE VAN AND SHARPENS MY KNIVES EVERY SIX MONTHS FOR A FIVER EACH; I JUST MAINTAIN THE EDGE HE MADE UNTIL IT REQUIRES HIS ATTENTION. THIS IS A HIGHLY RECOMMENDED APPROACH TO KNIFE MAINTENANCE IF YOU'RE A BUSY BEE LIKE ME, AND IT SUPPORTS THE LOCAL ECONOMY.

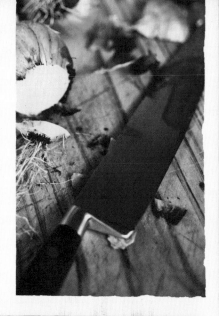

MEAT CLEAVERS

IT DOES ALL THE HARD WORK FOR ME. THE HEAVIER AND OLDER THE BETTER, ESPECIALLY IF YOUR DOING A LOT OF BUTCHERING YOURSELF. MY FAVORITE IS AN OLD, PORTUGUESE-MADE CLEAVER I BOUGHT OFF A BUTCHER. I HAD IT PROFESSIONALLY SHARPENED AND IT'S TURNED FROM ANTIQUE INTO A FORMIDABLE KITCHEN WEAPON.

HEAVY-BASED CUTTING BOARD

YOU CAN GET AWAY WITH ONE BUT TWO ARE BETTER: ONE TO BE USED FOR MEAT, AND ONE FOR VEGETABLES. HEAVY-BASED TIMBER WORKS WELL AND WILL PROVIDE STABILITY.

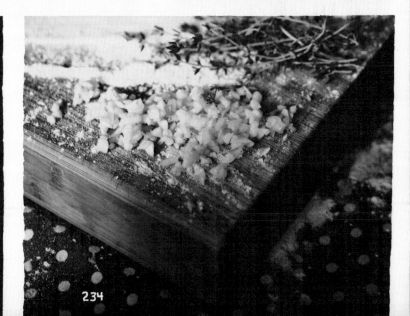

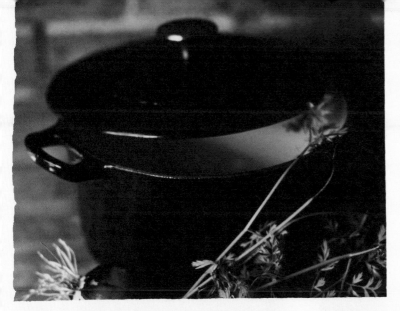

CAST IRON DISH

THEY CAN BE USED TO STOVE FRY, DEEP FRY, OVEN BAKE, AND SLOW STEW. ONE OF THE BEST PIECES OF KITCHEN EQUIPMENT I OWN. YOU CAN GET CHEAP ONES BUT THEY WON'T LAST AS LONG, SO SAVE UP AND GET SOMETHING THAT'S GOOD ENOUGH TO PASS DOWN TO THE NEXT GENERATION. SPEND AT LEAST $100 MINIMUM.

THICK BASE STAINLESS STEEL FRYPAN

YOU CAN GET THESE AT COMMERCIAL KITCHEN SUPPLY OUTLETS. WHAT'S GREAT ABOUT THEM IS THAT YOU CAN PLACE THEM STRAIGHT INTO THE OVEN, AND YOU CAN USE STRONGER KITCHEN IMPLEMENTS (AS OPPOSED TO THE SOFT-PLASTIC ONES REQUIRED FOR NON-STICK PANS). YOU CAN ALSO GET THIS TYPE OF FRYING PAN WITH LONG HANDLES, WHICH ARE GREAT IF YOU TAKE IT OUT FOR SOME CAMPFIRE COOKING!

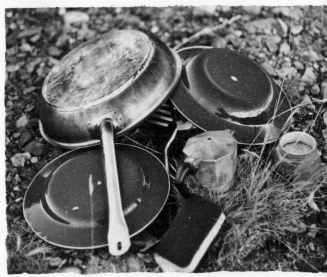

PESTLE AND MORTAR

THESE THINGS HAVE BEEN IN USE FOR THOUSANDS OF YEARS IN VARIOUS FORMS AND FOR GOOD REASON. THIS IS A VERY USEFUL AND OFTEN UTILIZED TOOL IN MY KITCHEN. GET THE MOST OUT OF YOUR HERBS WITH A LITTLE BASH TO RELEASE THE NATURAL OILS, OR EVEN TO MAKE THE MOST BASIC OF MARINADES, DRESSINGS, AND SPICE RUBS. ADDED BONUS... NO BATTERIES REQUIRED.

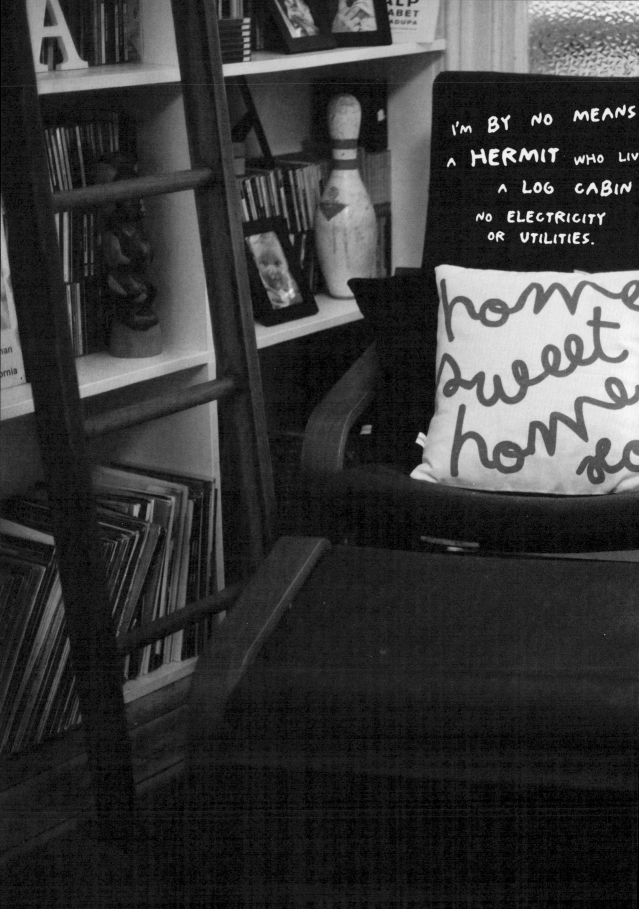

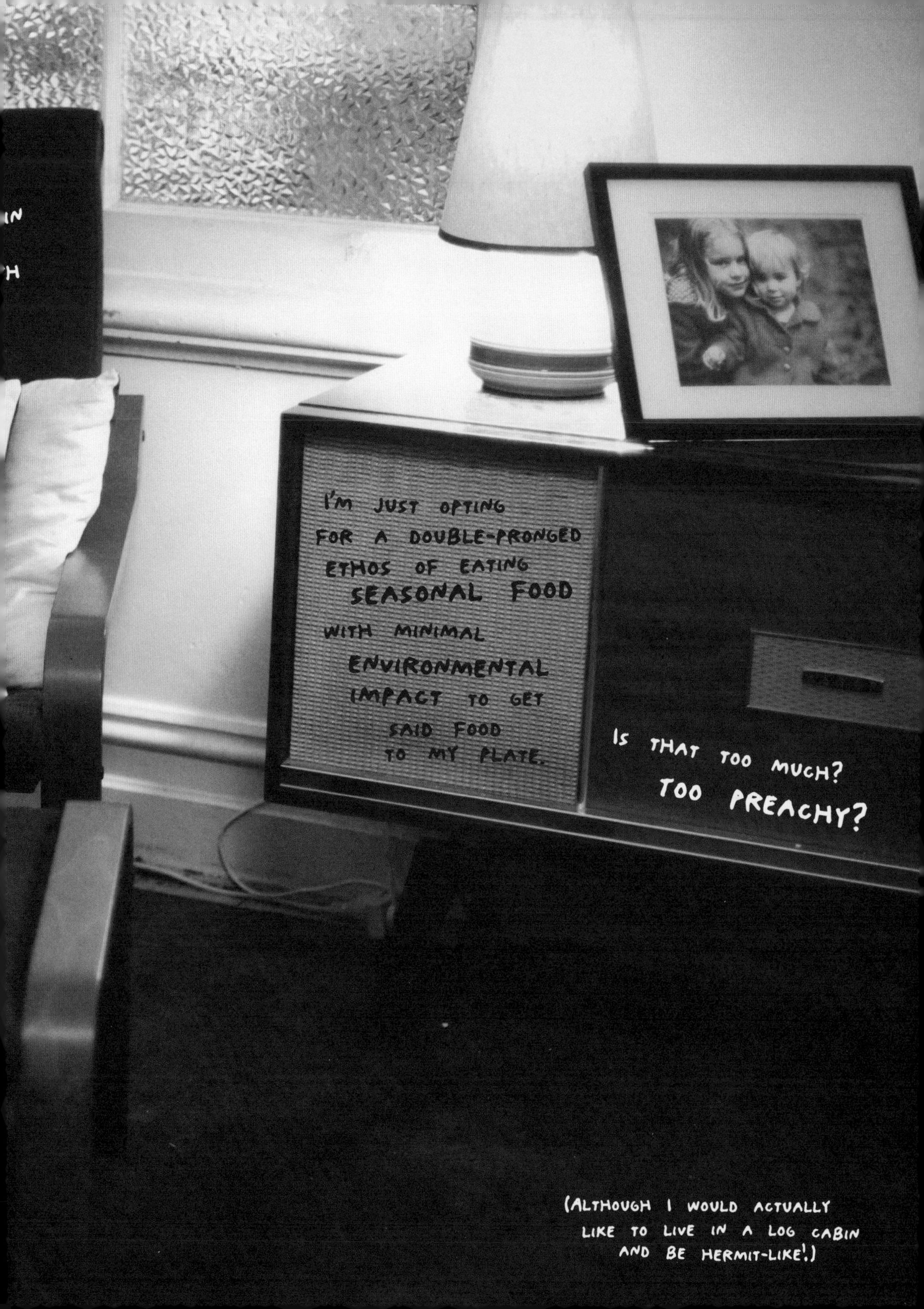

I'M JUST OPTING
FOR A DOUBLE-PRONGED
ETHOS OF EATING
SEASONAL FOOD

WITH MINIMAL
ENVIRONMENTAL
IMPACT TO GET
SAID FOOD
TO MY PLATE.

IS THAT TOO MUCH?
TOO PREACHY?

(ALTHOUGH I WOULD ACTUALLY
LIKE TO LIVE IN A LOG CABIN
AND BE HERMIT-LIKE!)

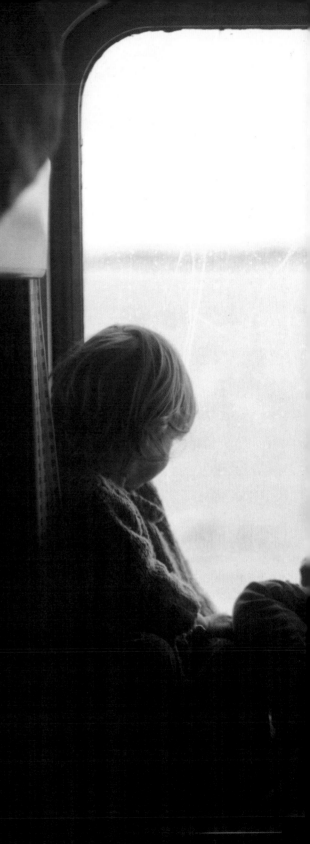

THE THANK YOU BIT:

A GREAT BIG THANK YOU
TO THOSE DEAR PEOPLE THAT
HAVE SUPPORTED (PUT UP WITH)
ME DURING THE PROCESS OF
MAKING THIS BOOK. NOTABLY
KIM, WHO BELIEVED IN ME
FOR SO LONG AND ENDURED
MANY A RABBIT DISH. THANK
YOU OLD FRIEND. A SINCERE
THANK YOU TO FRAN, WHO
SAW SOMETHING IN WHAT
I WAS DOING AND DECIDED
THAT I WAS WORTH INVESTING
TIME TO. THANK YOU TO
WILL LUCKMAN, WHO ASKED
ME TO WRITE THIS BOOK.
THANK YOU TO THE GUYS AT
POWERHOUSE BOOKS, CRAIG,
WES, NINA, AND MY DESIGNER
ERIC. THANKS CHRISTINE FOR
THE ILLUSTRATIONS.

THANKS TO EVERYONE ELSE
THAT HAS EITHER BELIEVED
IN ME, SUPPORTED ME, OR
INSPIRED ME AND IN SOME
WAY HELPED THIS PROJECT
HAPPEN; FOSTER HUNTINGTON,
JAMES FOX, JOAKIM SIMONSSON,
AMY MERRICK, CATH +
DREW, MATT BIRCH, JEFF
ADAIR, MARGARET BURIN +
ANDY, EMMA + JOEL, PETA
AMAZING, JUZ + SIMON, JACK
DICKINSON, PETER DEBICKI, LUCY
FEAGINS, PIP LINCOLNE, KATE
+ BREN, DEC + TORI, JOHN
PERGOLIS, KATE BERRY, AND
OF COURSE MY GIRLS HELENA
AND TIA AND MY PARENTS,
MUM AND DAD. MAD LOVE TO
YOU ALL.

XORO

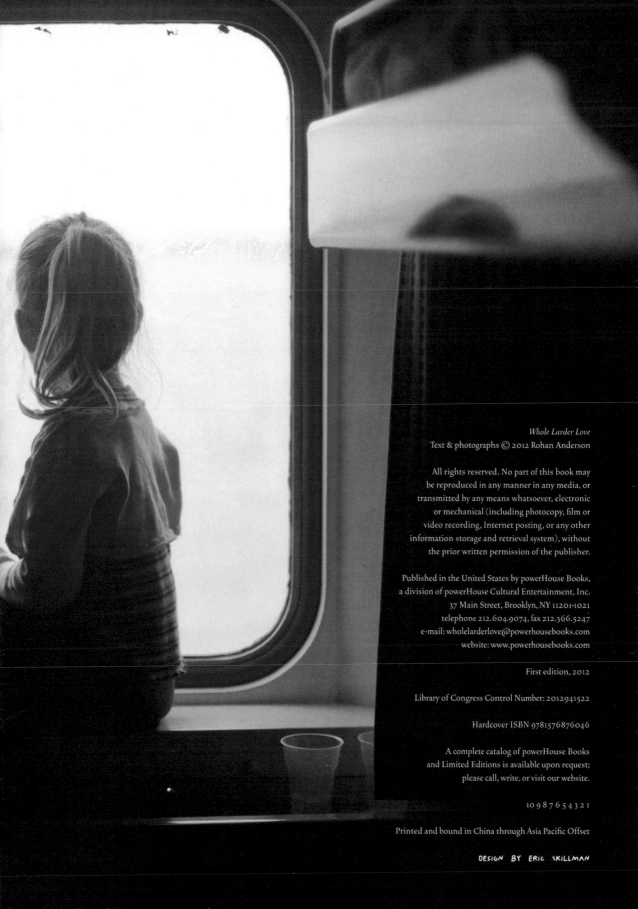

Whole Larder Love
Text & photographs © 2012 Rohan Anderson

Published in the United States by powerHouse Books,
a division of powerHouse Cultural Entertainment, Inc.
37 Main Street, Brooklyn, NY 11201-1021
telephone 212.604.9074, fax 212.366.5247
e-mail: wholelarderlove@powerhousebooks.com
website: www.powerhousebooks.com

First edition, 2012

Library of Congress Control Number: 2012941522

Hardcover ISBN 9781576876046

A complete catalog of powerHouse Books
and Limited Editions is available upon request;
please call, write, or visit our website.

10 9 8 7 6 5 4 3 2 1

Printed and bound in China through Asia Pacific Offset

DESIGN BY ERIC SKILLMAN

GUIDE TO THE GOOD LIFE

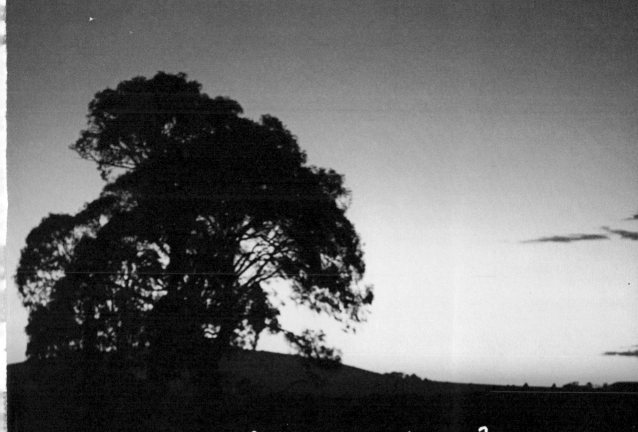

WHAT WAS ON TV TONIGHT...?

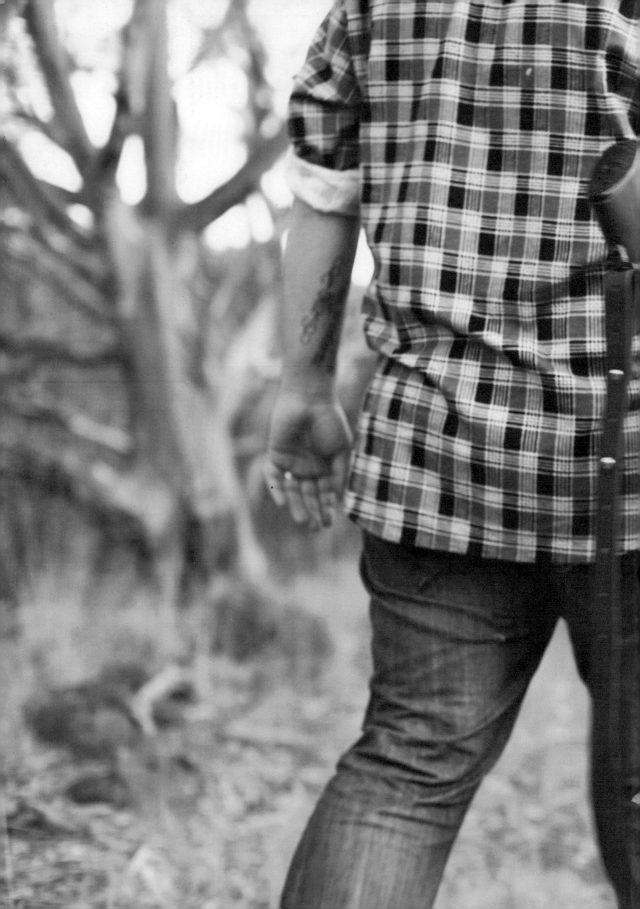